NATUROPATHIC
WISDM

A Common Sense Mind-Body Approach
for Struggling Children & Teens

Marlo Payne Thurman, PhD

NATUROPATHIC WISDOM
A Common Sense Mind-Body Approach for Struggling Children & Teens

All marketing and publishing rights guaranteed to and reserved by:

FUTURE HORIZONS

(817) 277-0727
(817) 277-2270 (fax)
E-mail: info@fhautism.com
www.fhautism.com

ISBN: 978-1-957984-73-5

CONTENTS

NATUROPATHIC WISDOM

— Chapter 4 —

— Chapter 5 —

— Chapter 6 —

CONTENTS

— Chapter 7 —

— Chapter 8 —

— Chapter 9 —

— Chapter 10 —

CONTENTS

— Chapter 14 —

— Chapter 15 —

— Chapter 16 —

— Chapter 17 —

Common-Sense Recommendations for Serious Mental Health Crises

PREFACE

When I began this work, I imagined telling stories, talking about my experiences, both personally and professionally, and connecting the things that I learned within my formal studies in naturopathy to my work in mental health. While I clearly attempted to stick to that script within the pages of this book, what I found most surprising throughout the writing process was how often I caught myself threading a fine needle through opposing and sometimes radically polarized points of view.

In today's world, we are divided and told that everything is either black or white; that there is a right position and a wrong position; and that healthy children are raised by parents with good values, the right political and religious affiliation, and 'proper' parenting methods. There is also the assumption that the increase we are seeing in mental health, learning, and behavior disorders in today's children and teens is created by the 'opposing side,' be that spiritual belief, political affiliation, or educational alignment.

NATUROPATHIC WISDOM

Moreover, and more than ever before in my lifetime, so many things that were openly discussed and shared in times past have now become flash points into political agendas. Even by bringing up certain topics, our positions are assumed, we are misunderstood, and we are judged, by one side or the other. Like most people my age, I have acquired some strong opinions about certain things that the reader might not agree with, as I am sure is a true statement for us all. But as you read this book, I hope you will recognize my attempt to honor all sides and positions in this work, and if what you read here offends you, please know that is ok. I only ask you to honestly consider my words, even if they do not at first ring true to you. Then, if you still disagree with me, great! Because if there is one truth that I embrace 100 percent it is this—there are as many good opinions about raising children as there are children, and we are all equally at a loss about what to do with the current state of 'unwellness' we see in so many of today's youth.

CHAPTER 1

Why Today's Kids Need Naturopathy

Chapter 1

Icame into the field of naturopathic medicine in the same way that many people do, through chronic illness that was not well treated through traditional western, allopathic medicine. But as is true for all individuals who suffer from long-standing illness, the years of my illness did not exist in isolation. Throughout my health crisis and as I moved into my own wellness journey, I also worked in the mental health field assessing and treating children and teens with learning, behavior, and mental health disorders. In the chapters ahead, I will share with you the insights I have gained across a thirty-year work history, as these evolved through my own personal health challenges. I will also detail solutions within alternative medicine and share my formal training in naturopathy. In so doing, I hope to offer some common-sense applications within naturopathy to address the needs of children and teens who are struggling. But before I go any further, let me clarify, I am an educator and mental health practitioner with doctoral-level training in School Psychology, Special Education, and Naturopathic Medicine. I am not a naturopathic physician. Within these degrees, I believe my work is best described within the terms of 'counselor,' 'consultant,' and 'educator' working within a 'naturopathic lens.'

So why does my background matter? In my profession I have been helping families and teachers with special needs children and teens for decades. This means that I have seen a lot of change in parenting and wellness practices through the years, and as I have watched recently, I have grown quite concerned. Today, far too many kids are not well, and the rate of mental illnesses and learning disabilities in children and teens is higher than it has been at any other point in recorded history.

The Rise in Learning, Mental Health, and Behavior Disorders

I began my work in the field of education and mental health in the late 1980s. At that time, childhood conditions such as Attention Deficit/Hyperactivity Disorder (ADHD), Autism Spectrum Disorder (ASD), Specific Learning Disorder (SLD), and the related mental health conditions of anxiety and depression were not that common in children. As an example, in 1989, autism alone was believed to affect only four of every 10,000 individuals (McMahon & Ritvo, 1989). Figures from 2021 indicate that the incidence of ASD is now approximately one in forty-four (Centers for Disease Control [CDC], 2021). While people can argue that the rate has increased, in part, due to better identification, as someone who has spent considerable time in the schools, I remember the days when there really were only one or two children with 'autistic-like' traits in an entire school district. Today, as I pass through the halls of most schools I visit, I see those traits in at least one or two children in every classroom. This alarming increase is also reported across other mental health, developmental, and learning conditions.

Research confirming my own observation for the rise in these disorders in our children is well documented. For example, in June of 2022, the Centers for Disease Control reported that in the United States, 9.8% (approximately 6 million) children ages three to seventeen were diagnosed with ADHD, 9.4% (approximately 5.8 million) children were diagnosed with anxiety, behavior disorders were diagnosed in 8.9% of all children (approximately 5.5 million), depression was diagnosed in 4.4% (approximately 2.7 million), and specific learning disorders occurred in 16.6% (approximately 10.3 million). While we all understand that children can be diagnosed with more than one of these conditions at the same time, and many children are multiply diagnosed, rough numbers still suggest that as many as 25% of all children nationwide carry at least one mental health, behavior, or learning disorder label. Even more shocking is this: 9.8% of all children in the U.S. aged five to seventeen take one or more psychotropic medications to treat a mental health or behavior disorder (CDC, 2022). Just for a moment let's really think about these statistics and ask this question: in all the written records across our entire human history, has there ever been mention of another time when one in four children were believed to be mentally ill or so significantly impaired in their ability to learn and develop that some treatment was required? Furthermore, isn't it concerning that one in every ten children take a medication that has a significant and often unknown impact on their development in cognitive and neurological maturation?

Changes Across the Past Fifty Years

During my lifetime, I have seen some dramatic changes in how children are raised, fed, and educated. Not surprisingly, in addition to my views on wellness, I also have strong opinions about what could and should be done differently from the standpoint of education and learning. But as I look today at both child-rearing practices and children's education, I think the most obvious change in my lifetime is this: as a society, we seem to have lost our most basic common sense about the natural relationship between physical wellness and mental health, and in so doing we've forgotten how interconnected we really are to the natural world around us.

As has always been true, children need healthy food, adequate sleep, plenty of fresh air and sunshine, and opportunities for physical work, play, and exercise. With these observations in mind and within the pages that follow, I intend to provide a basic, common-sense roadmap for the implementation of safe naturopathic practices that I believe

Chapter 1

are desperately needed for today's children. To cover these topics, I will use a method in formal research that is referred to as retrospective auto-ethnography. This simply means that I'll be looking back across my life to share my experiences and evolving beliefs. As I do this, I will focus primarily on what I think should be done immediately to improve the wellness of today's children and teens. More specifically, within the narrative of this work I will: 1) highlight relevant aspects of my own illness-to-wellness story that are applicable; 2) share professional observations and insights gained from my mental health practice of thirty-plus years; 3) propose simple, safe, naturopathic interventions for the physical and mental health conditions I see in today's children and teens; and 4) detail the research that supports these practices. As is common within all auto-ethnographies, I'll begin by briefly telling you a little about myself.

CHAPTER 2

My Story

Chapter 2

My story is not really that unusual. People my age usually have had an accident or two, a few major illnesses, and many of us are starting to really "feel our age" in ways that we never thought possible. But with all the negatives that the aging process brings, there are also nice positives. As we grow older, we become much less concerned about what others think, we stop trying to achieve accolades and accumulate "stuff," and for the first time, we truly become exactly who we are; we also begin the process of looking back, across our own lives, with a desire to share. So it is with the insights that have come from growing older, that I share my story.

Growing Up in Rural America in the 70s and 80s

I was lucky. I grew up in the 70s and 80s on a small family dairy farm in rural Wyoming. This matters because my family knew a little something about sustainable farming practices. As I consider my childhood now, I can see that my parents also often applied this same knowledge to what I will call "sustainable parenting." We ate nutritious food, lived in a clean and healthy home environment, got plenty of physical exercise in both our work and our play, spent lots of time outside where fresh air and sunshine were abundant, and we had a community of people looking out for our wellness. On the farm, we also lived close to and in deep harmony with the ground beneath our feet, and we were well versed in the life-giving abundance that the earth around us provided. When crops grew tall and we harvested them in season, we gave thanks and appreciated our blessings; when times were hard, we faced challenges together as family, friends, and neighbors.

Sadly, it was during the last years of my childhood that the rural dairy farms that had dotted the American land-scape for hundreds of years were subsidized and bought out nationwide, by commercial and government farming operations. So, by the time I left home to attend college, the farms and ranches of my childhood were all but gone. For me that meant there were no longer farm animals who doubled as family pets and few people still grew food in their own backyard. For America, this meant that most dairy products, meat, and food production farming had come under corpo-rate enterprise. I personally recall the first time my family bought milk from the store—it tasted empty and flat.

The Path Towards Poor Health

In 1986 I moved to 'the city' to attend college and there we ate poor-quality food, lived in cramped, noisy, and often unclean dorm-rooms where alcohol and drugs were abundant, and for those who did not play team sports, we got very little exercise. Called the 'freshman thirty,' I remember the upper classes making fun of us new students because we all gained weight. It was here that I started down my own path to poor health.

Transferring to an even larger and more demanding school for graduate studies, I began working with children who suffered from extreme physical, sexual, and emotional abuse. Here, I first witnessed the relationship between healthy children—what kids ate, their home environments, the opportunities they had to play outside—and the mental health and cognitive impairments that came from the absence of these. Yet, with over one hundred graduate school credits under my belt at that time, and with a focus that was always on child development, there wasn't a single class on children's eating habits, the effects of environmental toxins on cognition and learning, or even on the role that exercise plays in the developing child. While you might imagine that we obviously assumed these things, they were never discussed.

I still recall one girl specifically assigned to my treatment group who routinely came to the center in only her underpants, with lice and filth covering her entire body, even though we had bathed her at school the previous morning. This child was nothing but skin and bones and presented with both childhood schizophrenia and intellectual disabilities (her mother was also intellectually disabled). As her program progressed and the family began receiving food assistance, home supports, and training which included teaching the mom how to keep her home clean, feed the children properly, and basic safety and wellness coaching, this child's mental health disorder all but disappeared. She also gained 50 IQ points in less than six months. I will note here that in my training, neither low IQ nor childhood schizophrenia is a condition that should go away. But as I watched this child's remarkable transformation, which took less than six months, I began to understand how basic health and wellness underlies both physical and emotional health.

Trauma and Too Much Prescription Medication

After graduate school, with two young children of my own, I made the decision to start correcting my own poor eating and exercise habits, and for the first time since leaving my family home, I focused on 'getting healthy.' As is true for many 'starving graduate students' we had gotten through by cutting corners in both groceries and in time spent on wellness. So, at thirty years old, and across two pregnancies, my lifestyle choices were beginning to take their toll. It was during this time that my dad said this: what you save at the grocery store, you will spend many times over at the doctor's office. I knew these words were true, but

Chapter 2

I didn't get the chance to live them. Not long after that I was struck and injured by an 800-pound pallet of conference tables that fell from the shelf of a large garden-center warehouse. In this accident I sustained multiple injuries including a traumatic brain injury (TBI), and this pushed me deep into my reserves and well onto a long-lasting path of poor health.

Following my accident, and because I was suffering from the cognitive side effects of my TBI, which were making it difficult to work, various physicians placed me on a dozen different psychotropic medications in under one year. In eighteen months, these either contributed to or outright caused both partial and temporal-lobe seizures. My health worsened further as my doctors then tried to treat my seizures with even more medicine. By the time I stepped away from western medical treatments (a full fifteen years later), I had almost constant kidney and bladder infections, had suffered from full body hives for three years, continued to have seizures and black-outs many times per month (one that had caused a car accident in which I broke my neck and sustained a partial spinal cord injury leaving me barely able to walk), and I had been diagnosed with several autoimmune conditions, which came with both allergies and asthma. I also suffered from a complex range of gastrointestinal symptoms that occurred with most everything I ate. In fact, my allergic reactions to many foods and environmental toxins had grown so severe that

I carried two epi-pens to treat myself for allergy-related anaphylactic shock. In the end, I had even begun reacting to certain synthetic fabrics.

At forty-five years old, I was truly sick! I still have a few photos taken during those years, and in them, it is hard for people to even guess my age because my hair had thinned to less than 25 percent and had turned almost completely white. In addition, my skin was dry, thin, and gray, and I stooped and limped like an incredibly old woman. Maybe I am vain, but when my hair started falling out in clumps, I came to this conclusion—on my current path I was headed to an early grave. So, in a 'last-ditch' effort to save my own life, I made the decision to stop taking all my various medications (I am not recommending this for anyone) and solve my health problems myself. Although I almost died from this journey, I did eventually start down a road towards alternative and integrative medicine that would finally heal me in both mind and body.

Finding Alternative Treatments

During the last few years of my illness and as I began a quest to find alternative methods of treatment, I also got truly lucky because my work in the field of autism introduced me to a small handful of the world's best biomedical doctors. Let me back up a moment. In graduate school, I had started working with kids with autism and by the time I was in my mid-thirties, I had been asked to join the advisory board for the US Autism Association (I'm now their president and board chairman). It was here that I was introduced to alternative medicine under the labels of 'functional,' 'alternative,' 'nutritional,' and 'biomedical' as these fields were emerging to treat some of the more challenging symptoms of autism spectrum disorders.

Within my work in autism, and given my own state of advanced illness, these 'autism doctors' became beacons in the dark for me, as it was through them that I gained enough hope and confidence to start the long journey towards healing my own body. By sitting in on training sessions offered by these specialist physicians, for the first time in my life, I began to fully understand how deeply integrated the mind and the body really are. Within this discovery, I learned also that I could treat the seizures that had plagued me for over a decade through basic detoxification and wellness practices and with the use of strain-specific cannabinoid oils. I also discovered that all my seemingly distinct health conditions, which required various specialists and physicians to treat, were rooted, at their most basic level, in my poor, underlying physical health. This may seem obvious, but as both a very sick patient and a professionally trained mental health practitioner, before this time in my life, I had truly never been taught to think about the deep co-relationships that occur between physical wellness, the array of my diagnosed medical conditions such as asthma, allergies, digestive issues, etc., and their ties to mental health.

In fact, across all the countless doctors that I had seen in a roughly fifteen-year history of treatment, not one had ever inquired about my diet or nutritional practices, my basic exercise and wellness routines, or even about my sleep. I'll add here that it was also during the final years of my illness that I returned to graduate school to obtain a Ph.D. in Special Education. Even here, in another degree specifically focusing on child development, there still was not a single class on health and wellness in an entire doctoral-level curriculum.

The Division of Mind and Body in the Treatment of Illness

Just so you understand how separated mental health and physical health were, and still are even today, I will share an interesting side story. During a lawsuit pertaining to my brain injury in 1999, my case made national history for 'being the first case in the U.S. in which a plaintiff was able to prove that as an organ of the body the brain can be injured' (Denver Post, 2000). In fact, my lawyer won 'Trial Lawyer of the Year' for making the case that the brain is not necessarily subject to the $250,000 statute of limitations, which had previously been set forth in the courts as the maximum lawsuit amount for patients with a mental health condition. In a five-day jury trial, this portion of the case took over four hours to deliberate, in a packed courtroom. Sadly, I am not kidding.

Unfortunately for many childhood conditions, especially in autism (which is the childhood disorder that I am most familiar with), there still seems to be little recognition for the physical health conditions that commonly occur beside or beneath various mental health disorders. For example, did you know that just last year depression was found to be closely aligned with inflammation and diet (Chen, Faris, Bragazzi, 2021)? But except in extremely small circles, having certain conditions such as depression or autism doesn't bring about improved medical care. In fact, these diagnoses can even become a reason to *assess no further* for far too many diagnosed individuals. To this day, only a small handful of specialty trained physicians exist to treat mental health within a more holistic and wellness-based lens. But those that have training in both western allopathic medicine and in more non-traditional, eastern, functional, or biomedical medicine are still at risk of upsetting the 'medical establishment' in the U.S. and legally losing their licenses. In fact, I have a good friend who recently lost his medical license for refusing to refill opioid prescriptions and instead proposing alternative treatments such as vitamin-B injections, the use of hyperbaric oxygen chambers, and heavy metal detoxification.

NATUROPATHIC WISDOM

The Road Back to Health and Wellness

You might find it interesting to know that my story does eventually have a happier ending. Working often on my own, and occasionally with the limited help of exceptionally rare, unique, and alternative medicine practitioners, I finally discovered how to stop my seizures. I also found the underlying cause of my severe allergic reactions, and through genetic testing, I discovered and treated my "histamine switch;" I also healed my gut. Last, with severe joint, nerve, and arthritic pain in nearly every part of my body, I finally stopped taking prescription pain pills, replacing these with herbal remedies., and I got myself moving (I now swim sixty laps three to four times per week). Today, I still have a spinal cord injury. I also need to be quite careful with my diet, especially when life's stressors become high, as I occasionally can get a few hives (which are now simply a good reminder for me that I am falling off track). But it has been over a decade since I had my last seizure, I no longer have any allergy or asthma symptoms, and I can honestly attest to the fact that for the first time in at least twenty years, I feel like I am getting younger and not older, and I take only one medication to treat my low thyroid condition.

For me, the combination of naturopathic, alternative, and biomedical treatments did not work overnight; it took a lot of time and effort on my part to figure things out, often through both trial and error. Thankfully, I was also able to

Chapter 2

fall back onto the healthy, sustainable, lifestyle foundations that I had grown up with. In the end, I did heal my body and my mind through healthy eating, exercise, and basic wellness habits. As I did this, I realized that my health had been off the rails for many years, and poor lifestyle practices for me were combined with severe injury, secondary illnesses, and far too many prescription drugs. But some of my doctors were also to blame because they paid little attention to treating my whole-body system. In hindsight, I can now clearly see that without a complete, mind-body-wellness approach, I would have never gotten better, and I may have even died. For me, a major lifestyle change was necessary; yet not a single doctor I worked with recognized or promoted those changes.

Shared Experiences

As I began to heal, I also started seeing how much of what I was learning about myself related to what I was seeing in my clients. This forced me to really start examining wellness in the mental health arena. Finally, at the age of forty-nine, I made the decision to formally pursue studies within the field of naturopathic medicine. It was here that my own wellness journey evolved alongside that of my professional studies to forever change my views on mental health and wellness in my clients. This ultimately shaped the treatment model I use today. This work is the culmination of my journey.

I will add here: **this book is not intended to, nor should it be misconstrued as medical advice.** Furthermore, **I am not a licensed naturopathic doctor.** What worked for me, or for one of my clients might not work at all for someone else. But in this book, I have chosen to share with you what I feel are the most logical and commonsense wellness practices that I believe can and should be implemented for every child, and especially for those with special needs. I will close this chapter by saying this: if I have done my job well in authoring this book, what you read here should ring true to you, and the information within these pages should simply sound like basic common sense. Because in the end, I believe common-sense is exactly what the field of naturopathy intends for us to learn.

For those who want to understand the specific research methodology used in this work, the following section briefly explains that aspect.

CHAPTER 3

Research Methods & Perspectives

Chapter 3

Within research methods, there are essentially two basic types of inquiries; these are referred to as either qualitative or quantitative. Quantitative studies are the studies that we hear the most about, because these include the random clinical trials used by pharmaceutical companies, the medical research community, and the large opinion polls and population studies that provide data about everything from our shopping preferences to who is predicted to be our next president. While these types of studies make up a substantial portion of research inquiries, qualitative studies are important as well. While quantitative studies give us small bites of information across large groups of people, qualitative studies give us a larger and more in-depth understanding about certain conditions or situations because they specifically explore the ways in which the people who have lived with these conditions or situations have learned from their experiences (Merriam & Tisdell, 2015).

In my various graduate programs, I have done both qualitative and quantitative research, and I have a doctoral minor in statistics, which helps me in interpreting quantitative research. But for this project, I specifically chose a qualitative methodology to examine, in depth, my own changing thoughts, perceptions, insights, and beliefs across my personal and professional life, for the purpose of giving others a new way to think about the topic of wellness for today's children.

The Role of the Researcher in Auto-Ethnography

I first began to think about the relationships between physical and mental health when I saw my first truly mentally ill child over thirty years ago. Since then, I have wrestled with unresolved questions about why, as a society, we do so little to teach parents and professionals about mind-body health and wellness. Throughout my career, I have seen approximately 3,500 children, all referred for various special needs. In my opinion, not one with true mental illness has been healthy in the physical sense.

Within qualitative inquiries, the researcher becomes the primary research instrument for the study (Merriam, 1998). In the beginning of my fifteen-year battle with severe illness, I believed that my experiences with illness, injury, and subsequent mental health disorder were unique, that I was an exception to the norm. But as I began to see myself through the lens of the children in my mental health practice, I also began to see that so many of the children I worked with were far more like me than they were different, especially within their physical and mental health relationships, even though the stories for how these children had become ill were of course very different. On multiple medications, these children too had dark circles under their eyes, looked pale, had no energy, complained of stomach and digestive issues, had blotchy skin, and suffered from allergies, illness, and autoimmune conditions. As was also true for me, these physical symptoms were largely ignored.

My Lens as a Researcher

Over time, my perspective about the relationship between mind and body wellness changed and evolved, and as I lived my life and practiced mental health professionally, the two perspectives merged. For those who like to have the formal research terms named, this process in qualitative research is referred to as the building of a *social and historical constructionist's worldview* (Burr, 2003). In lay terms, this simply means that my worldviews evolved out of the merger between my own experiences with illness, within the social relationships that I had developed through the years with my doctors and various mental health professional and educators, and through my interactions with the clients in my practice and their families. In looking back, it was clearly within these relationships, that I *constructed* my opinions and beliefs, and these guided me towards formal studies in the field of Naturopathic Medicine.

I think I have also always been curious to understand and construct meaning about why children become mentally ill. I have also always wanted to know what more can be done to treat these conditions. Qualitative researchers Trochim and Donnelly (2001) add that within most qualitative studies, the life-long interests and curiosities of the researcher ultimately result in the emerging perspectives of the research. I truly believe we can only know and understand the world from the position of our own reality and through our own lived experiences. From there, as we share our stories with others, we arrive at our own sense of meaning. In the field of qualitative inquiry, according to Blaikie (2007), this makes me a *realist*. Within this worldview, personal *knowing* is an inductive, bottom-up position that comes from observing the world, then constructing and creating theories about how things are related to each other. It is then within the sharing and testing of theories about what we think and understand as these relate to the views and beliefs of others that we create meaning. Within this worldview, true knowledge only emerges when it is shared and evaluated against the experiences of others, with every individual developing their own thoughts, feelings, and beliefs across a lifetime.

In summary and for those looking for my formal research methodology statement, this work is a *qualitative research inquiry*, written in the form of a *retrospective autoethnography*, which is framed in *social constructionism*, with the conclusions interpreted through an *inductive, realist* lens.

Chapter 3

All that said, whether you're a research scientist or the parent, teacher, or mental health clinician for a child or teen who is really struggling, I believe that the method I chose for this work helped me to describe, understand, and share my impressions about why so many of today's children and teens are being diagnosed with learning, behavior, or mental health illnesses. This retrospective auto-ethnography also provides detailed information about what can be done to better address wellness needs within basic principles of naturopathy. Using this approach, the work provides a commonsense road map and a 'best practices guide' supporting the inclusion of basic naturo-pathic practices into discussions and treatments to better to raise, educate, and address mental health, learning, and behavior in today's youth.

CHAPTER 4

What Exactly Is Naturopathy?

Chapter 4

When I began my doctoral studies in naturopathy, I was not even exactly sure what the word naturopathy meant. Back then, I had a basic understanding that it related, in some vague way, to alternative medicine, and that herbal medicine was included. But in truth, in the beginning, I lacked even the most rudimentary understanding about the wide range of therapeutic practices that traditionally fall under the umbrella of naturopathic medicine. Assuming there are others who, like me, need a foundation before we can really talk about naturopathy for its application to raising children and teens, I will first tell you how naturopathy is defined. From there, I will share an abbreviated history about the field of naturopathy as it evolved alongside traditional western medicine. Last, I will provide information about the core values and beliefs that usually align with or have full inclusion under the umbrella of naturopathic medicine.

Primary Elements in Naturopathy

In my studies, I've come to understand that the primary elements in naturopathy, in fact the very keys for both physical healing and mental health and wellness for the naturopathic practitioner, include: 1) fresh clean air; 2) pure water; 3) safe and sensible exposure to the healing benefits of the sun; 3) nutritious, high-quality food; 4) adequate and restorative down time, rest, and sleep; 5) and vigorous physical work and exercise (Paulien, 1995). Most naturopaths also include hydrotherapy, massage, acupressure, and plant-based healing within their naturopathic practices. For me personally, a sustainable and healthy relationship with myself, with others, and with the planet is also required for proper healing and wellness within a naturopathic lens. I'll add that when an individual is in harmony within their body, which is the goal of the naturopathic healer, there often also comes a deepened sense of self, purpose, and belonging to a world that is created and sustained by a *positive and loving divine force*. While other naturopaths may define things a bit differently for themselves, I'll wager that almost anyone who considers themselves a naturopathic practitioner holds these keys as central to their own lifestyle choices and uses these daily within their chosen career path as a naturopathic healer.

Within these keys, there is the belief that in most circumstances, and in the absence of severe bodily injury, the body knows how to heal itself—that there is some natural blueprint within our very code for survival for wellness. Thus, if given the right circumstances, most illnesses and injuries resolve naturally and on their own, within a full return to healthy and sustainable living practices. Given these underlying assumptions, the naturopath views poor health and disease, primarily from the perspective of poor life and health style choices. Starting here, the healing journey begins only by returning the body to its best state of balance and wellness. Thus, within a truly holistic system of healing, the naturopath strives to bring into harmony an integrated wellness of mind, body, and spirit through simple, healthy, wholesome living (Shelton, 1895).

Spiritual Nature of the Naturopathic Practitioner

Because the naturopath sees the healing journey as one of whole, mind-body wellness, it should not, therefore, be a surprise that most naturopathic healers also tend to be more spiritual than those working in other healing traditions. Because of this, when I refer my clients to naturopathic or alternative/biomedical practitioners, or even integrative medical practitioners (traditional doctors working within a more holistic lens), while religious affiliation and spirituality are often subjects not openly discussed in other fields of medicine or mental health, I've learned to *warn* parents who are not familiar with naturopathy to expect a higher than usual degree of spirituality within the practitioners that they will encounter. In my clients, this quick 'heads up' is often enough to prevent the families I refer from being thrown off by spiritual, divine, or God-based statements or iconography in discussions, websites, or in the offices of naturopathic practitioners.

I'm not alone in recognizing a correlation between spirituality and naturopathy. In a large clinical study conducted in 2009, researchers Farr, Curlin, Rasinski found that when compared to traditional medical doctors, doctors practicing naturopathy, complementary, and/or alternative medical interventions were three times more likely to refer to themselves as "very spiritual," even though their rates of participation in formal religion were not necessarily that different from those reported by traditional physicians. To me this means that within the very definition of a naturopathic treatment model, it helps to know that practitioners tend to be more closely aligned to their own version of spirituality.

Personally, especially as I have dug deeper into understanding the remarkable healing benefits of the millions of plants that grow on the earth, it has become impossible for me to believe that a world so abundant with healing plants that literally grow right out of the ground beneath our feet, could ever have existed if there wasn't some higher power involved in the earth's creation. While I have not always been deeply religious, the more I study this field, the more spiritual I have become.

As my own growing understanding about the complexities and unknowns of earth-based wellness for the body has evolved, I am also reminded of a quote by Dr. Charles

Chapter 4

Sherrington, the grandfather of modern-day neurophysiology, in his discussions about the intricacies of the mind. He describes the mind like this: *an enchanted loom where millions of flashing shuttles weave a pattern meaningful though never abiding, it is as if the Milky Way has entered in upon itself in some cosmic dance* (Sherrington, as cited in Hansotia, 2003).

To me this means that the human body, the mind, the planet on which we live, and the vast cosmos around us are still far from being understood. This also suggests the possibility, as first proposed by Armstrong (2010), that the miraculous and biodiverse cosmos and the physical world that surrounds us is mirrored within the neurodiversity and complexity of the human mind and body. Thus, with what are likely to be astoundingly complex and interrelated systems, there are still then millions upon millions of unknown relationships between the human mind, our physical bodies, and the healing aspects of our life-sustaining planet that we still have not yet discovered.

Core Principles of Practice for the Medically Trained Naturopathic Doctor

With so much left to learn, the core principles that have been accepted for all naturopathic medical providers, as detailed by the Association of Accredited Naturopathic Medical Colleges (AANMC), and as accepted by most other naturopathic practitioners at all levels of naturopathic training, are agreed upon as follows:

First Do No Harm

Core to all medical practice is the desire to help the human form and condition. NDs typically approach care by utilizing the most natural, least invasive, and least toxic therapies. NDs refer to other physicians when the patient's presentation is outside their scope or level of skill.

The Healing Power of Nature

NDs recognize the value of our natural world in assisting the healing process. Not only do NDs utilize substances that originate in nature, but they also incorporate a healthy natural environment as foundational to human health. Naturopathic doctors recognize and harness the body's inherent wisdom to heal itself in order to guide patients to wellness and total health.

Identify and Treat the Causes

There is a time and place for symptom suppression. However, most naturopathic patients will benefit from identifying the underlying causes of illness and removing obstacles to cure.

Chapter 4

Doctor as Teacher

Naturopathic doctors elevate patient health literacy. That means that NDs are part of the team helping patients have a better understanding of what it takes to be and stay well. Through education and a trust-based relationship, patients better understand the steps they need to take to achieve and maintain health.

Treat the Whole Person

Naturopathic doctors understand the interconnectedness of our body, our environment, and our lifestyle on total health. It is only through this whole-person-based approach that NDs seek to restore balance and health.

Prevention

Naturopathic medicine affirms that it is better to prevent illness and suffering whenever possible. Through their comprehensive practice, NDs combine all six principles in order to identify potential areas of imbalance and teach patients how to get well and stay well.

(AANMC, 2022)

CHAPTER 5

The History of Modern-Day Naturopathy

Chapter 5

It has been said that naturopathy is the "oldest healing system in the world" (Sharps, 1995, p. 1). Throughout history, the various practices of healing have all, necessarily, relied heavily on 'letting nature take its course,' because in so many cases, that was all we could do. As defined within the Merriam-Webster online dictionary (2022), letting nature take its course literally means "to allow something to happen without trying to control it as in the injury should heal within a few weeks if you just *"let nature take its course."* With similar healing traditions present across many different societies worldwide, the sick and injured have historically been treated through the years with basic home remedies. Then, when additional care was needed, barber-surgeons, local folk healers, shamans, and conjurers (Newson, 2006) administered treatment. It is only within the past one hundred years that licensed physicians have solely prevailed within the field of medicine.

While botanical medicine (the use of plants and herbs to treat illness and disease) predates recorded history, written records suggest that the use of botanicals goes back to at least 5000 A.D. when the Mesopotamians recorded their use of plant-based medicine on clay tablets (Pan, 2014). With these records still visible today, and with the benefits of these early findings now verified within modern-day scientific studies, it is safe to assume that botanical medicine has been used, with varying degrees of effectiveness, through-out our human history.

Through the dark and middle-ages, medical knowledge, at least throughout many of the major European countries, was carried forward primarily by religious orders such as the Benedictine Monasteries, who copied ancient medical texts, saving them for posterity (Medeiros & de Albuquerque, 2012). But with monasteries serving as the primary medical treatment centers of their day, it is not known how much of what the monks who copied the ancient texts actually understood or properly applied to their care of patients; we do know that the monasteries did have some remarkable herb gardens that have been described in detail in multiple records, however.

Most historians agree that the evolution of medicine changed most dramatically when the Black Death of the seventeenth century raged untouched by the standard medical practices of that time. Purging, sweating, bleeding, blistering, and vomiting, along with the use of purgatives, emetics, opium, cinchona bark, camphor, potassium nitrate and mercury were standard practices in medicine back then (Parascandola, 1976). It was during these years too that formal medical training, which primarily included lessons in anatomy and dissection, also became requirements for those practicing medicine. But, with formal training in place, healers also became more sharply divided between those who practiced the 'old natural ways' and those who practiced

Chapter 5

within the 'new scientific methods' of medicine (Fee, 2015). This put into motion a pendulum that pulled those who were sick between allopathic, 'science-based' practitioners and those without formal training who employed 'ancient, tried-and-true' methods that had been promoted throughout much of human history.

The Birthplace of Modern-Day Naturopathy

Thus, with practices that are potentially as old as man, for our purposes, and to gain a deeper understanding about how modern-day naturopathy was formally established and defined, we'll pick up the division between the 'scientific' doctors of the 1800s and the earth-based healers of that era in the year 1895. It was in this year that the term "naturopathy" was originally coined by John Scheel who then later sold the term to Benedict Lust, the Father of Modern-Day Naturopathic Medicine. In that same year however, Lust credited his training to Germany's Father Sebastian Kneipp, who was a strong advocate for 'the drugless method' of treatment for illnesses and disease. Father Kneipp developed a treatment method that was referred to as the Kneipp Cure. Like Kneipp, Lust promoted exercise, diet, manipulative therapies such as massage and acupressure, herbs, hydrotherapy, homeopathy, and emotional rest within his formal definition for the field naturopathy (Cody, 2018).

NATUROPATHIC WISDOM

Dr. Kneipp's own story is a fascinating one, as it was during his lifetime that the pendulum between the old nature-based ways and the new scientific brand of medicine of that time took a hard swing, for some, away from the modern medical practices of the time. This opened the door for the emergence of the field of naturopathy that we now recognize today (Ko, 2016). Kneipp was a weaver's son who had fallen ill with a life-threatening disease and instead of being treated by the physicians of the day, cured himself. From there, he began to treat others within the methods that had worked for him, and as his reputation as a healer grew, his methods were made available to rich and poor alike, with Kneipp even treating the Roman Catholic pope at one point. Over time, and with an ever-increasing number of healing testimonies supporting his work, Kneipp became an international celebrity who today is credited for single-handedly turning his small farming village into a "world-famous spa" that treated tens of thousands from all over the world. Kneipp is best known for reminding the medical establishment that there was still value in the basic healing practices of nature-based cures (Locher & Pforr, 2014).

Following in the tradition of his mentor Kneipp, according to Czeranko (2019), Benedict Lust organized the fledging movement of Naturopathy, rallied Naturopaths across America to practice according to the laws of Nature, established one of the earliest health food stores in America, opened the first Naturopathic College, and presided over the American Naturopathic Association throughout his life. In so doing, naturopathy as we know it was firmly established.

Medicine in the 1800s

To more fully understand the factors that led to Kneipp's success, and to the emergence of our modern-day naturopathy, during the final years of the 1800s, it is also helpful to consider what was occurring at that same time within 'scientific' medical practices. During most of these years, under the 'Miasma Theory of Disease,' it was still widely accepted that illness was caused by some imbalance or disturbance within the body that was brought on by things like foul odors in the air, evil spirits, some contagion, or any number of bad external influences (Ajesh, 2018).

It is also notable that physicians practicing during these years, as had been true since 400. B.C. when first proposed by Hippocrates, accepted the belief that to cure disease, one must eliminate bad and often external influences that had taken up residency in the body. This was done through the cleansing or releasing of blood, yellow bile, black bile, and phlegm, which were referred to as the four humors (Lagay, 2022). Thus, the physician's role was to release these influences through the practices of bloodletting and by actively 'chasing out' the offending influence through the mouth, nose, pores of the skin, or the rectum with the assistance of various purgatives.

But according to Bordley and McGehee (1976), it was during the mid- to late 1800s, when Kneipp's work was in its heyday, that the traditional medical practices of the trained, 'scientific physicians had become particularly bold and aggressive.' During these years, practitioners were all but abandoning the older procedures of cupping and bleeding and had moved towards increasingly more dangerous purgative and stimulant drugs including cocaine, heroin, lead, and even arsenic. Combined with the rise of the 'traveling doctor' selling all manner of 'snake oils' and 'poisons,' going to a modern-day doctor during these years had become a truly risky business (Stromberg, 2013).

Changing Times and the
Germ Theory of Medicine

But like it has done since the earliest traditions of medical practice, the pendulum continued to swing, and even with a revived interest in more natural and drugless healing approaches formally emerging and becoming popularized in the late 1800s and early 1900s, the pendulum was also pulling back towards science-based medicine within the work of microbiologist Louis Pasteur (Smith, 2012).

Chapter 5

In fact, by the time that naturopathy was officially emerging as a worldwide trend, Pasteur had already become a household name for discovering that by killing off certain bacterium in food, a wide variety of digestive illnesses could be circumvented. From there, Pasteur identified and eradicated a specific microorganism that was killing silkworms, and this led him to propose his "germ theory," which by the early 1900s fully shifted the cause of many diseases away from 'unknown external forces' to that of microorganisms now capable of being seen with a microscope (Britannica, 2021).

Pasteur actually began his work in 1878 when he developed a way to vaccinate chickens and other farm animals suffering from bacterial diseases. Under the belief that by giving the animals a small amount of the bacteria, in a weakened form, one could introduce the animal to the illness for the purpose of building immunity, human vaccines emerged. But even with Pasteur's advances in science and medicine changing forever the way people viewed foodborne illnesses and illnesses in animals, it was not until well after the turn of the century that the medical establishment fully embraced the 'germ theory of disease' for use with humans.

NATUROPATHIC WISDOM

The Rising Powers of the
American Medical Association

Once beliefs shifted away from unknown and external causes for disease and toward new views on treating visible germs, bacterium, and viruses, licensed medical professionals of the day, under the growing power of the American Medical Association (AMA), moved toward aggressively stamping out all medical practices not approved within their organization (Baer, 2001). Calling their own work 'regular medicine' and the work of everyone else 'irregular,' for the first time in history, the AMA became a policing agency actively tracking down and incarcerating healers practicing folk medicine, naturopathy, and even basic chiropractic care (Cody, 2018).

By the 1940s, the AMA fully controlled all licensing laws regarding who could legally practice medicine. With powers to practice medicine in the United States granted by the federal government, the AMA also claimed regulatory control over all activities related to health care. In this way, organized 'allopathic' medicine gained full control over health care and segregated out those individuals practicing homeopathic, naturopathic, and osteopathic medicine. In his description of the remarkable change of power in medical treatments for the sick that occurred in only a few short decades in the first half of the 20th Century, Paul Starr (2004) states:

Chapter 5

From a relatively weak, traditional profession of minor economic significance, medicine [became] a sprawling system of hospitals, clinics, health plans, insurance companies, and myriad other organizations employing a vast labor force. This transformation has not been propelled solely by the advance of science and the satisfaction of human needs. The history of medicine has been written as an epic of progress, but it is also a tale of social and economic conflict over the emergence of new hierarchies of power and authority, new markets, and new conditions of belief and experience.

Medical and Mental Health Horrors of the 1900s

With rising oversight and control by the AMA resulting in indisputable gains in medicine during these years, it is also beneficial to remember that during the same years the AMA was incarcerating naturopaths, it also endorsed a fair number of 'regular' medical practices that are considered barbaric by today's standards. A few of these endorsed practices include: the drinking of radium water; the treatment of cysts, hemorrhoids, and other 'unwanted bodily protrusions with ecraser (using a metal loop that was increasingly tightened until a particular unwanted part of the body lost enough blood to rot and fall off); the use of plombage in which those suffering from ailments of the lung would have the bottom portion of their lungs surgically filled with foreign matter, such as small, lucite balls; the administration of morphine and surgical lancing of babies' gums to treat teething pain; the use of mercury, arsenic and deliberate inoculation of malaria to treat syphilis; and the use of hydroelectric (electroconvulsive) baths for the treatment of everything from erectile dysfunction and headaches to severe mental illness (Holland, 2019).

In fact, by 1950, within the rising power of the AMA, and due to politicization of the 'germ theory' which associated germs with poverty, race, and even religious beliefs, the door flew open for both forced sterilization and lobotomization, especially for certain poor, minority, and mentally disadvantaged groups (March & Goloso, 2020). Notably between 1949 and 1950, 65,000 people were lobotomized in the United States alone, with the youngest of these being only six years old (Faria, 2013). I will pause here and ask you to really think about the support and power that the medical field held at that time. In so doing I'll also ask—under what circumstances would we now let anyone simply dig around inside another person's head with an ice pick or other sharp surgical tool? I've specifically chosen these few examples to demonstrate how far at least some physicians had strayed from natural, common-sense healing methods in medicine by the late 1950s.

Chapter 5

The Ever-Swinging Pendulum

With some of these atrocities in mind, a civil rights movement that was in full force, and with a war overseas that was not well-supported by many Americans, by the late 1960s the pendulum moved again. It was during these years that individuals rebelled against many traditional Western establishments in the U.S. by taking their cases to court. This resulted in major shifts in civil rights for the individual, which once again included the right to engage in the services of alternative, naturopathic, and even chiropractic treatments (Snider & Zeff, 2019). It was also within these counter-culture movements that the various practices defined in the late 1800s in naturopathy once again became more widely practiced and were re-popularized. This meant that as had been true before, the general population once again embraced working within the more natural lens that the field of naturopathy provided. During the mid-1970s in particular, hydrotherapy (in the form of bath houses), herbology, and various home-based remedies became especially popular.

In the past fifty years, the ever-increasing focus on hard science within the allopathic/western medicine model has continued to clash with those continuing to practice alternative, biomedical, and naturopathic medicine. The most notable evidence of these clashes since the 1970s has been seen within the various vaccine debates (Wolfe & Sharp,

2002). In fact, in just the past three years (and with the emergence of the COVID-19 pandemic), the AMA has proposed mandatory vaccines for all illnesses that significantly affect public health (Shachar & Reiss, 2020).

But within this movement, alternative, biomedical, and naturopathic practitioners have sided with informed consent proponents and remained in support of an individual's right to choose, in all circumstances, when making personal health care choices; this includes getting vaccinated. So, this question, like so many others of the past, has sharply divided and polarized the nation.

It is within this continuum of divide that I suspect the pendulum between allopathic and naturopathic treatments will continue to swing well into the future. It is also within this very swing that one day, a balance between science and the nature-based practices of our ancestors may eventually be reached.

In the meantime, and in addition to a divided nation on a wide number of medical topics, we are also seeing sharp differences between these two groups about what should constitute adequate training and professional licensure for individuals who call themselves Naturopathic Doctors. Within these divisions, most states are moving towards requiring all naturopathic providers to be licensed by the AMA, with even those offering basic coaching in exercise, wellness, and nutrition being called upon to attend medical school. In time, this move may prove to be a good thing, or

Chapter 5

it may be another example where the pendulum swung too far. But in either case, as has been true since the term naturopathy was first formally coined and detailed, the field of naturopathic healing continues to hold true to its original standards of treating the sick through basic, common-sense wellness practices established eons ago.

CHAPTER 6

Health & Wellness in Today's Youth

Chapter 6

With an increased understanding about the mind and over 100 psychiatric drugs available to treat various mental health conditions today, I'd love to be able to say that I believe the current state-of-affairs for treating mental health, behavior, and learning disabilities in children and teens is much better than it was a hundred years ago. I would at least like to say it is better than it was in the 50s, when kids with learning, behavior, or mental health disorders ran the risk of being sterilized or lobotomized. But for some of the clients I see in my practice, unfortunately I am not so sure.

Positive Changes in Mental Health and Education in the Past Fifty Years

I will start off by saying I have witnessed profoundly positive changes in the ways that those with severe mental health are treated in just my lifetime. When I was in my early twenties, my first opportunity to work with individuals with severe mental health and behavior needs was in a residential group home for individuals identified as needing significant support due to their autism.

During a Reagan-Era move toward deinstitutionalization, the group home that I was hired to assist in managing was slated to accept the last five (and most severe) children and young adults still residing in the Utah State Hospital system. To prepare the home for the care of these severely affected individuals, I was recruited to tour the state-run facility. In my one-hour tour, I saw children shackled to their beds; individuals so heavily medicated that they couldn't speak, wake, or close their mouths; and living quarters that while reasonably clean and sterile, still reminded me a bit too much of the horrifying Geraldo Rivera undercover documentary *Willow Brook: The Last Great Disgrace* that was filmed in 1972. With almost all of these state facilities closed, we now have community-based treatment homes to meet the needs of these individuals, and at least some of these are exceptional.

In the field of education, I've also seen many positive advances as I've been blessed to be able to advocate for individual student needs under the Individuals with Disabilities Act of 1990, which gave all children the right to a free and appropriate public education; under the No Child Left Behind Act of 2001, which added significant changes for accountability in schools for all children; and under the Every Child Succeeds Act of 2015, which increased educational transparency and reporting about student growth in learning. Compared to the years when disabled children were simply kept home from school, the positive progress in education is commendable.

Chapter 6

Recent Trends that Concern Me

But with all these good changes, I have also seen some bad. In today's schools, children are more heavily 'tracked' for their academic and behavioral performance than they have ever been before. Added to this, because school funding is now deeply reliant on children's performance scores, for most, this trend has resulted in even more pressure for teachers and children to perform. For children who naturally succeed, core standards have certainly increased learning outcomes and improved overall academic performance. But for children who learn less traditionally or learn on their own developmental clock, and for those who cannot easily manage the stressors of 'high stakes' performance standards, the result seems to also include a significant rise in diagnosed mental health disorders. Being a kid in today's schools is no easy feat!

Furthermore, for kids who do not fit in and/or who can't keep up, which I see rising in number each year, the standard reaction by both schools and parents has been to refer more and more children for mental health therapies and psychopharmacological treatments (Racine, et al. 2021). This trend became even worse during the COVID-19 pandemic (Theberath et al., 2022). Between 2020 and 2021, I personally watched as those who had learning styles that were not well matched to online learning failed their classes, many for the first time ever. I also saw that far too many of my off-beat, quirky teens, did not return to school once lockdowns were reversed—these kids simply stayed home from school because staying home had become their norm.

While a small percentage of kids did better during the COVID-19 pandemic, because of highly motivated parents who had the time and financial resources to build for their children something better than what traditional school offered, for the majority of kids who are now in trouble, online learning practices placed many students behind, and made it difficult or even impossible for some to return to regular school. This has now resulted in large numbers of kids becoming what I call 'couch-locked' due to failed classes, an inability to graduate with peers, and ever-increasing degrees of low self-esteem combined with poor physical and mental health. In today's world there are far too many teens and young adults who are so completely disenfranchised with their schooling and with normal life that suicidal ideation is also at an all-time high.

The Rise in Psychotropic Medications and Possible Long-Term Repercussions

Within these concerning mental health trends, there unfortunately is still little being done to integrate what seems like 'basic wellness practices' into the educational and home-life routines of today's youth. In fact, within both the fields of mental health and medicine there are still almost no discussions about nutrition, fitness, and the overall wellness needs that I believe underlie the very physical, cognitive, and emotional challenges that today's kids are now facing. I also see far too many families resigned to letting their kids entertain themselves online, across all hours of the day and night.

In addition, and in a trend that seemed to begin in the mid- to late 1990s and worsened dramatically in the past three years, I've also seen increasingly large numbers of children who regularly take prescription medications (sometimes several different ones at a time) to treat what I consider to be 'questionable' mental health conditions. It seems to me that kids who live their lives mostly online, with irregular sleep schedules, virtually absent of exercise and proper nutrition, and with no normal social exposure to the world, should be treated first and foremost for their health and wellness and for 'online addiction.' Only then should these kids receive treatment with medications for their residual mental health symptoms, because truly little is known about what the effects of the rise in these medications will be in future years on developing brains and bodies.

Through the years, and because many of my clients tend to stay in contact with me, I've watched as children and teens from the past who took multiple prescription medications in their youth moved into adulthood; these young adults now seem to be suffering from an unusually higher than average amount of physical illness along with continuing and debilitating mental health conditions. While my observations are drawn from a small sample size of only several hundred kids, it seems that despite their severity as children, those who were heavily medicated tend to fare much worse as young adults than those who dealt with their mental health or behavioral conditions without the use of medications.

Mental Health Diagnoses Used as a Reason to Not Treat Physical Symptoms

As a final concerning trend, I have personally also witnessed that children with mental health diagnoses often are not properly treated for their medical conditions. Even more concerning, I've seen that the mere presence of a mental health diagnosis can prevent proper medical treatment, especially for those with more serious mental health and behavioral conditions.

To give you an example, about three years ago I saw a child referred for paranoia, anxiety, and depression who did not have regular bowel movements. In the bout of constipation that brought him to my practice, he had not had a bowel movement for sixteen days when his primary care physician again agreed to see him for constipation (he had been seen several times before). At this meeting with his medical doctor, and with the symptoms of the child reported

Chapter 6

as excruciating agony when going to the bathroom, this boy and his parents were told by their physician to 'go home and see a therapist' to 'get over the boy's fear of defecation.'

This boy was luckily referred to me for assistance with his 'irrational fears' and for support in treating what his physician believed was paranoia over going to the toilet. His condition was not surprisingly accompanied by anxiety and depression. Let's stop right there for a moment. Can you imagine as an adult being seen by a doctor for an inability to pass feces, then being blamed, shamed, and sent home to suffer? I saw this boy for only one session and immediately referred him to a good integrative medicine doctor that I often work with. There, his bowels were irrigated, he was assessed for allergies and food sensitivities (and was found to have several), and he was treated for an inflamed bowel through dietary support and nutritional counseling. After dramatic dietary changes, he was also placed on a special strain of probiotics that helped him normalize his digestive system. In less than four months, this boy's paranoid symptoms, anxiety, feelings of sadness, and suicidal ideation were fully resolved, as were his digestive issues.

With this story and countless others like it in mind, I can personally attest to the fact that many children with diagnosed mental health conditions are routinely denied proper medical care. To me, it is just common sense to say that if a child cannot go to the bathroom and is storing feces in the intestines and lower bowel for weeks on end, there are obviously physical conditions that should be addressed before treating the child for a mental health disorder. But for children with autism, certain severe behavior disorders, or significant mental illness, in my observations, reported symptoms are frequently ignored and interpreted instead through the lens of the mental health condition. This means that for these children, diagnosis of their mental health or behavior disorders unfortunately results in less not more physical health care.

Today's Kids are Not the Same Kids

I have been seeing kids since 1987. In these years there have been unexplained increases in the rates of autism, ADHD, and in the number of seriously suicidal teens. I have also personally witnessed the emergence of more complex learning disabilities, and in the children and teens I have assessed, I have also observed a noticeably widening gap between their cognitive strengths and weaknesses on even the most basic IQ tests. Both anxiety and depression are also at an all-time high in children and teens, and like you, I have stood by as silent witness to more teen and young adult mass shootings than we can even now remember or count.

This leads me to ask: what is happening with today's youth? I suspect that there are many different variables. But as someone who has worked with kids, and specifically

Chapter 6

focused on those with learning, mental health, and behavior disorders for over thirty years, I'm here to tell you this: **many of today's kids are not the same kids that I saw less than twenty years ago.** These kids are vastly different in ways that I cannot easily explain. In addition to what I see in their learning and behavior, today's kids are far more prone to food allergies and sensitivities, problems with strength and physical stamina, and lack basic resilience and cognitive energy. If you look at these kids carefully, many also appear physically sick, with sallow skin, dark circles under their eyes, thin dry hair, and poor standing and sitting posture. Something is very wrong with far too many of today's kids, at the most fundamental health and wellness level and I would really like to know what is causing this. I would also like to know if in today's mental health and educational systems we are properly identifying and treating mental health and learning conditions. Moreover, with our arsenal of options in psychopharmacology, I would also like to ask this: are we doing more harm than good in the treatment of mental health, learning, and behavior disorders when the conditions we see in children and teens are not well understood for their underlying physical wellness causes?

With so many reasons to be concerned about the health and wellness of today's children, it seems simple to me that the inclusion of basic wellness practices, as these are defined within the field of modern-day naturopathy certainly cannot make things worse. In the chapters that follow, I will detail these practices, along with the research supporting them, and I will include my experiences, thoughts, and recommendations from a personal lens to share how I think the concerns detailed above should be addressed. Before I detail these practices though, it is important to provide you with some basic information about choosing a naturopathic practitioner.

CHAPTER 7

Choosing a Naturopathic Practicioner

Chapter 7

Unlike Western Medicine Doctors (also referred to here as Allopathic Doctors), Naturopathic Doctors are not consistently trained throughout the U.S. within core standards or specific degrees of clinical experience. This means that some doctors who practice naturopathy are fully trained physicians that attended medical school, while other naturopathic doctors may be 'self-taught.' With such a massive range of training and skill level in this area, I think it's important for us to spend a few minutes discussing the various levels of training and certification that might be found in the various practitioners that call themselves Naturopathic Doctors. I will add here that many chiropractors also refer to themselves as naturopathic doctors.

State-Based Differences in Licensing for the Naturopathic Doctor

In a basic online search conducted in October of 2022, all states across the U.S. now fall into three categories for licensure status for practitioners working as Naturopathic Doctors. These include: 1) states that require traditional medical school training, board licensing exams, and an official state license to practice; 2) states that offer (but do not require) licenses where a variety of different degrees, licenses, and certificates are able to practice legally based on various court cases, with or without license; and 3) states that neither license nor offer licensure for individuals to refer to themselves as naturopathic doctors (within this category some states have made it illegal to deliver any form of naturopathic service). But even within these core distinctions, each state has specific criteria that can be found within the states' Department of Regulatory Agencies (American Naturopathic Certification Board, 2022, October 8).

To begin this discussion, it is initially helpful to know that across all states where individuals are allowed to practice naturopathic medicine, naturopathic providers cannot write for prescription medications and cannot perform medical procedures or surgeries that require the use of anesthesia without holding a full medical license.

Training, Certification, and Licensing Differences

Across states that allow the practice of naturopathy without attendance in medical school, there are varying degrees of training along with several 'accreditation' and 'certification' licenses that mean quite different things. For example, the program from which I graduated (IIOM) is accredited by the American Naturopathic Medical Accreditation Board

Chapter 7

(ANMAB), and by the American Association of Drugless Practitioners (AADP). These are two of the major boards offering training guidelines and accreditation for distance-learning schools to offer formal training in naturopathy. Within these accrediting agencies, doctoral-level candidates can 'sit for licensing' in certain states to become 'Board Certified.'

But these Board Certificates do not necessarily allow practitioners to work as naturopathic practitioners in most other states, and the majority of states are now moving towards a full, medical-school licensure model for all persons practicing naturopathic medicine. In these licensing states, no person is allowed to refer to themselves as a 'Naturopathic Doctor' without completion of a four-year medical-school training program that is accredited by the Council on Naturopathic Medical Education (CNME). Candidates in these programs must not only attend medical school alongside of other allopathic medical students, but they must also complete a minimum of 4,100 hours of in-person clinical work under the supervision of a licensed naturopathic medical doctor before they are eligible to sit for examination on the Naturopathic Physicians Licensing Exam (NPLEX). Once licensed, these practitioners can practice as medical physicians, with certain limitations set for what they can and cannot do.

In 'fully licensed' states, lesser-trained individuals can still refer to themselves as 'naturopaths,' but they cannot charge money to offer even the most basic suggestions about lifestyle or healthy living choices without licensure in some other area, such as counseling. In licensing states, the use of 'ND' in the post-nominal letters of a person's professional signature byline is also prohibited.

Within partial licensing or alternative licensing states, the requirements vary so dramatically that these cannot be easily encapsulated in this discussion. But the first step to understanding licensing in each individual state is to determine which category, of the three categories listed above, the state falls into. From there, more specific research can reveal what training and licensure an individual practitioner must hold to practice. Last, state guidelines determine what licensed naturopathic practitioners can legally do; these are detailed within the state's regulatory board for naturopathic practice.

Should All Naturopaths Go to Medical School?

Let us recall that, within the modern-day field of naturopathy, as it was officially established over 125 years ago, practitioners have held firm to the belief that good common sense and sound health and wellness coaching and support should be freely shared by anyone who has the proper knowledge to do so. Within the naturopathic tradition, it is also widely held that naturopaths hold and carry forward a historical body of knowledge that has been not only 'cast out' but 'intentionally lost' within traditional allopathic medicine. So today, many of the individuals trained in naturopathy strongly oppose the state-based 'fully licensed mandates' that are sweeping the country at this time. These concerns stem from the fact that by attending medical school, the entire field of naturopathy could be indoctrinated and forever altered within a traditional, Western Medicine lens.

That said, as states argue to regulate and standardize professional business practices for the safety of the consumer, each state cites its own cases where individuals with no formal training in medicine, who referred to themselves as naturopaths, have sold medical services and caused harm or even death to those paying for their services. But even with the presence of these cases, it is interesting to note that the American Medical Association has credited the field of naturopathy for successfully treating chronic conditions that do not respond well to traditional medicine in certain cases (AMA Position Statement-Complementary Medicine, 2018).

Know Your States Rules When Choosing a Naturopathic Practitioner

So, like everything else in a divided world, my advice is this: before you work with anyone calling themselves

NATUROPATHIC WISDOM

a Naturopathic Doctor, Herbalist, Alternative Medicine Doctor, Biomedical Doctor, Functional Medicine Doctor, or Integrative Medical Practitioner please take the time to understand the training and licensing requirements under which the person is working in your state. Also, **do your research** about the credentials and training of the person with whom you are working.

I will add—personally, I do not believe that all good naturopaths are licensed physicians. In fact, some of the individuals who helped me the most on my healing journey were not licensed doctors at all. But I am saying that unlike most state-approved professional service providers, the services of a naturopathic provider can be wildly disparate, state-to-state, so it is up to you, the consumer, to know exactly what services you are paying for and if the services you are receiving are legal and reputable in your state.

Furthermore, please know that while there are some highly skilled naturopaths, both with and without formal medical school degrees, and many of these can and do share a wealth of information for sound healing practices that can't easily be found anywhere else, there are also some 'true quacks' out there who are calling themselves Naturopathic Doctors but really should not be allowed to perform any medical or wellness services. Also, as is true for treatment with all forms of care, either allopathic or naturopathic, use good common sense, trust your gut, and when things don't feel clear or right to you, ask questions, and

Chapter 7

get a second opinion. Also know that there is not anything at all wrong with finding a middle ground between allopathic and naturopathic medicine. This middle-of-the-road position is now usually called Integrative Medicine, and for many of my clients, that 'sweet spot in the middle' has been the most beneficial.

CHAPTER 8

Children Need
to Move

Chapter 8

Less than forty-five years ago, with few television channels, no internet, and computers that were viewed as 'fun toys of science,' children played outside. We ran races, rode our bikes, jumped rope, and climbed trees in the summer; and in the winter, we went sledding, built snowmen, and created elaborate snow forts. Thus, we were exposed, year around, to the outside world that included both fresh air and sunshine. On the farm, we also worked hard physically, using our bodies for the manual labor of carrying or dragging feed, cleaning cattle stalls, and changing out bedding for the animals. When time permitted, we also played, often as hard as we worked, hauling, stacking, and building forts out of heavy hay bales. In addition to our outside work and play, most kids our age also participated on one or more sporting teams and/or had other physical hobbies; we also had jobs outside of the home by the time we were sixteen or seventeen years old. Because our schools knew we needed to work to help out at home, homework from school took far less time than it does today. At day's end, we were truly tired in both mind and body, and for our generation, at least when we were children or adolescents, sleep was rarely reported as a problem.

NATUROPATHIC WISDOM

Movement As a Necessity for a
Healthy Mind-Body Interface

Today, according to several large national studies, children and teens spend the majority of their waking time indoors, either watching television or sitting behind a computer (Stiglic & Viner, 2019). Research beginning over ten years ago suggested that the typical Amercian child of the twenty-first century engages, on average, in less than 2.5 hours per week of physical activity, and this includes the time spent in a school gym class (Smith 2010). This time obviously decreased further as children went online for their learning during the COVID-19 pandemic, with most children during the pandemic receiving less than one hour per week of physical activity (Bates et al., 2021).

With such a massive change in children's outside and physical activity time across the past two decades, and even more dramatic decreases in physical activity in only the past few years, I've asked this question: how has such a major shift in the ways that children and adolsecents spend their time affected their physical, mental, behavioral, and emotional health? Think about this. Today's child is the first child in human history that is both educated and entertained, primarily while sitting or lying down.

It is well understood that children need physical play, as well as regular, rigorous exercise in which they must physicallyexert themeselves to develop a healthy

Chapter 8

mind-body interface. Let me explain why. Irrespective of our individual differences, all living beings must find a way to successfully access, integrate, filter, process, and organize the vast array of sensory information that comes in from the external world.

At the most basic level, an effective interface between the physical body and the world, through the system of sensory processing, dictates one's very capacity for learning and survival. But according to researchers Buzan and Buzan (1993), this mind-body interface works continuously and in constant relationship to everything that the body is doing and with the information provided from everything that is going on outside of the body in the surrounding environment. Thus, working simultaneously from the inside out, as well as from the outside in, the mind-body system is extraordinarily complex and integrates itself in non-linearity.

Let's pause for one moment and really think about what that means. To receive accurate information from the world outside of our bodies, one must essentially 'tune' multiple sensory receptors to the perfect frequency for the moment, then 'calibrate' the brain's systems of attention and arousal to locate a 'station' that is interesting but not stress producing. A 'frequency' that is too stimulating will create a stress response, and one that is too dull will go undetected. Next, the system of executive functioning must also 'attenuate' its sensors to the tasks of filtering, regulating, organizing, prioritizing, and relaying information. Once all of that has occurred, only then can a child pass any necessary or meaningful information forward for higher cognitive processing. Now, consider that all of this happens in a nanosecond with over one hundred billion brain cells simultaneously connecting to tens of thousuand of other cells (Buzan & Buzan, 1993).

Thus, when we take all of this into account, is it any wonder that some children cannot effectively process everything that the world around them has to offer? Now consider how the development of these systems changes when a child has little exposure to the world. According to Jean Ayers, who was a neuroscientist and the founder of the

field of Occupational Therapy, some children inherently struggle with the neurological process that organizes the sensations between the body and the environment. But others lack opportunities to develop. Either way, when the sensory system does not develop normally, it becomes impossible for a child to use their body effectively within the environment (Ayers, 1972).

Ayers adds that when this mind-body interface does not match up and develop normally, learning, mental health, and behavior in children will be significantly altered. In her work, Ayers specifically proposed that 'neurological breakdown' arises from an underdeveloped mind-body interface because of the 'miscues that occur at the higher centers of the brain.' According to Ayers, the child with poor mind-body connection will be unable to integrate, modulate, and properly interpret or react to incoming information (Schaff & Miller, 2005). Ayers' original theory addressed the five primary senses (touch, sound, sight, taste, and smell), but also incorporated the sensations of movement and pressure (DiMatties & Sammons, 2003).

With the goal to get kids moving in ways that would help them to develop a more normal mind-body interface, Ayers adopted the view that the everyday experiences of motion, movement, work, play, and deep physical exertion were the best ways to naturally integrate and develop these responses. Within this belief, Ayers created the field of Occupational Therapy to essentially get kids moving.

Research on Movement, Mental Health, and Learning

Since Ayers published her first paper on sensory processing in children, researchers have explored the relationships between movement and the mental and physical wellness of children. Several notable studies supporting the benefits of movement for child development include: 1) Castelli, Hillman, Bucks, and Erwin (2007) who directly correlated physical activity to academic achievement and found that children who were more sedentary have greater challenges with learning; 2) a large epidemiology study conducted by Boyle et al. in 2011 through the Centers for Disease Control that found increases in learning, developmental and mental health disorders were directly correlated to the amount of time that children spent playing outside; 3) a landmark study in 1997 by Aron and Aron that tied ineffective sensory processing to the diagnosis of anxiety disorders in children; 4) an Eysenck and Calvo (1997) study that aligned sedentary lifestyles with anxiety, and with one's ability to store and process new information within the working memory system; 5) and a final study by Lambourne, Audiffren, and Tomporowski (2010) showing that only 30-45 minutes of daily exercise significantly improves attention, organization, executive functioning, and learning.

Given these reports, it appears clear that physical exercise and movement do, in fact, help to integrate a child's mind-body interface. Movement decreases anxiety, improves sensory processing, aids in the cognitive tasks of memory and executive functioning, and decreases the rates of diagnosis for learning, mental health, and behavior disorders in children. To me, it does not then seem surprising that there is also a direct and clear correlation between the decreasing levels of movement in today's children and teens and the rise in their diagnosed learning, behavior, and mental health disorders.

Chapter 8

A Call to Get Kids Moving

Within the past ten years, and exacerbated in 2020 and 2021 when mandatory, at home, online learning for most children become the norm, we saw dramatic changes in the wellness of our kids. In fact, because these changes were so strikingly different than what was being reported in any other period over the past one hundred years, various child advocacy groups requested that the U.S. government call for a National Mental Health Emergency for Children and Teens. While we can only speculate that this mental health crisis aligned with the increasingly sedentary activities in both learning and play, there is certainly correlation to suggest such a relationship.

In my mind, given all that is known about the relationships between physical activity, mental health, and wellness, it seems obvious that if we want to reverse the mental health crisis in our youth, we must first strive to find better ways for children and teens to reclaim safe spaces to run, jump, play, socialize, and exercise. We must also re-examine the role that movement and physical activity have within learning. For many of my clients, I will add that team sports have not been a particularly good answer. So in my recommendations about movement, I frequently suggest daily time, outside, in a park or playground; fully enclosed outdoor trampolines and other safe playground equipment for use at home when kids need to jump, bounce, or work out their frustrations; scheduled weekly appointments in recreation centers and gyms to use climbing walls, swimming pools, and, as kids get older, weight rooms; individual competitive sports such as martial arts or swimming; and if necessary, occupational therapists, personal trainers, and fitness coaches when kids can't regulate their movements or sensory responses and/or when kids won't get moving on their own.

CHAPTER 9

Safe, Sensible Sunshine

Chapter 9

I believe that the best place to get kids moving is within the great outdoors. But as we have become increasingly concerned about ultraviolet radiation and the damages of sun exposure, it seems to me that at least within certain circles, the pendulum may again have swung too far in keeping kids indoors. For some of the clients I see, there is the assumption that all sun exposure is bad sun exposure. Added to trends for more sedentary learning and compounded by primarily indoor/online entertainment and socialization activities, many kids today really do not ever see the sun at all.

Sunshine Exposure in My Childhood

When we were kids, we did not wear sunscreen. In fact, in the late 80s, as teens, we intentionally bared our bodies to the sun to get a 'suntan,' using baby oil and sometimes even tinfoil, directed at certain areas, to speed up the tanning process. We also suffered from sunburns, complete with blisters and peeling skin when we had gotten too much sun, and as we have aged, we now must carefully monitor our skin tags, discolorations, and moles for the presence of skin cancer. We also get cataracts by the time we are in our late 50s or early 60s, and these too are blamed on unprotected exposure to the ultraviolet rays of the sun.

So, I cannot say if our years of exposure to full sun with no sunscreen were good for us. I can say that the sun's rays seemed much less intense back then. Whether this is due to rising ozone levels or whether we were simply better equipped to manage the sun due to constant and increasing exposure with better reactions in our melatonin (tanning) abilities is not clear. But either way, we could usually stay outside all day, every day, and not really burn after the first few days. For one summer, I was even an outdoor lifeguard with five to seven hours per day of sun exposure. Even then, I did not wear sunscreen. Now, for me, a single hour in the sun seems to cause the same burn that decades ago took a full day at the pool to acquire.

Historically, it was not until the early to mid-1990s that we all really started slathering ourselves and our kids with sunscreen. Today, I am certainly an advocate of not burning, and therefore, using at least some form of sun protection. But I still wonder what happened between the years of my childhood and prior and the years of today as kids have become increasingly protected from the sun.

Chapter 9

Sun Exposure: What the Research Tells Us

We do know that too much sun exposure can cause everything from a painful sunburn to deadly forms of skin cancer (Watson & Maguire-Eisen, 2016). But in defense of the sun, I would also like to share a few studies on sun exposure that I think relate to the topics of this book.

First off, most of us already know that exposure to the sun gives us a natural production vehicle for Vitamin D. But why is Vitamin D so important? Can't we just take a Vitamin D supplement? According to Wacker and Holick (2013), while most research says yes, a vitamin form is fine, vitamins might not be as effective as the actual sun in giving us Vitamin D and here's why. Naturally produced Vitamin D is created when the sun's energy turns a chemical in our skin, a certain cholesterol, into Vitamin D. From there, this form of the vitamin is carried to the liver and kidneys, where it is converted into active vitamin D. In its active form, Vitamin D allows our bodies to draw from our calcium and phosphorous stores for use toward healthy bone growth and maintenance. But active Vitamin D is not only used by our bones. According to Sirajudeen, Shah, Menhali, (2019) many other body tissues also have Vitamin D receptors (proteins that attach to the active Vitamin D), and researchers are only now just beginning to understand how Vitamin D affects these other places in our bodies where receptor sites exist. This means that while we still don't understand how the intestines, prostate, heart, blood vessels, muscles, and even endocrine glands, which all have Vitamin D receptors react to the sun, according to Aranow (2011), we do know that good things happen throughout the body when there is enough active Vitamin D in the body to bind to these receptors.

We also know that morning and midday sun exposure improves sleep by regulating and normalizing the timing and production of melatonin (Blume, Garbazza & Spitschan, 2019). This seems important for today's kids because without exposure to full sun during the day, the brain takes the next brightest light period of the day to alter melatonin production. What if that time of day is late at night, when kids are doing homework or winding down by sitting in front of a big screen television or computer, which also exposes them to full spectrum UV light? You guessed it, the body decreases melatonin at the exact time that it should be actively boosting melatonin for sleep.

Sun exposure also dramatically reduces stress hormones and lowers our reactivity to stressful events (Dhabhar, 2018). This means that being in the sun makes us more resilient to stress. This is also why, according to the Sunlight Institute, exposure to the sun between the hours of 8 A.M. and noon has been proven to help with regulating blood sugar and, in turn, speeding up weight loss (Mead, 2008). In other studies, regular, safe exposure to the sun also strengthens the immune system (Mullin & Dobs, 2007).

Chapter 9

For reasons that we do not yet fully understand, natural sunlight is also quite effective in treating depression. While this area is well researched, and many individuals world-wide suffer from the effects of Seasonal Affective Disorder (SADS), which is a specific form of depression that occurs during the lower sun exposure months of the winter, it is still not known what the full effects of sun exposure are on our mental health and wellness, or even why sun exposure is an effective treatment for SADS. What we do know is that SADS is not well treated with Vitamin D supplementation.

Of all the sun exposure studies I looked at though, the most interesting was a large, longitudinal study, where data was collected across three decades and included more than 30,000 people. This study found that those who reported seeking "regular sun exposure" lived, on average, 5.7 years longer than their matched comparisons who reported "I tried to stay out of the sun." This remained true even when all other variables, such as death by cancer, had been accounted for.

Is Sunscreen Really That Safe?

With hundreds of studies clearly supporting the health risks of too much sun exposure, along with numerous recent studies proposing cancer-causing health risks associated with several chemicals found in most sunscreens (MacMillan,

2022), are we better off today than we were in the days of our ancestors who did not have or use sunscreen? I know I personally cannot wear most sunscreens. These cause me to develop hives. I have also been quite concerned watching children as their parents spray them down with high UV protection aerosol sunscreens; many kids inhale these. This has caused me to ask this question: how safe is aerosol sunscreen when inside the lungs? With the safe use of at least certain types of sunscreens still unclear to me, and with both health and wellness benefits, and health problems caused by sun exposure, I'll share with you my thoughts about the sun, from my own life experiences, my understanding about how the sun helps us, and as viewed from the lens of naturopathy.

Recommendations for Safe Sun and UV Light Exposure

First, we all need to be outside, in the sun, for at least short periods of time each week. The best times for exposure to the sun are logically in the early morning or early evening when the sun's UV rays are at their lowest levels. I also recommend that children be protected from sunburn and from the damaging effects of the sun by wearing hats and clothing instead of sunscreen, whenever this is possible.

Chapter 9

When sunscreen is needed, I recommend that it be used in the lowest level of protection recommended, not the highest. I also believe that children should be prevented from inhaling sunscreen that is sprayed from aerosol cans. For children with sensitive skin, I have found that there are major differences in sunscreen brands, even within those with the same SPF protection. When sunscreen is necessary, I suggest finding 'sensitive skin brands that do not irritate the child's skin.

Additionally, it is my firm belief that children who are struggling to sleep at night should be exposed to natural sunlight in the morning, and if necessary, periodically throughout the day, even if only for a few minutes at a time, to establish good circadian rhythms and for proper regulation of the production of melatonin. As is also recommended by my good friend, Dr. Rebecca Hutchins, who is a pediatric optometrist, when children must engage with full-spectrum light at night, either from a television or from the full-spectrum light of a computer screen, blue-blocking eyeglasses can be worn to help the brain find a more natural 'twilight' level of light before sleep.

Last, it is incredibly important for parents to control bedroom lighting, the nighttime use of cell phones, computers, and TV screens. I believe that sleeping spaces should be dark enough to prevent the light pollution that disrupts melatonin production. This means that even small flashing lights from game controllers and/or flickering UV lights should be removed from sleeping quarters.

For children who cannot wake up in the morning, natural light can also be introduced incrementally to help. I have used various gradual-waking brands of alarm clocks and have found that the introduction of both light and sound, at increasingly intense levels, really helps some kids with waking.

CHAPTER 10

Breath Responses & the Air We Breathe

Chapter 10

I meet some utterly amazing people in my line of work. One individual that I had the pleasure of interviewing last year is a recognized expert in what is referred to as the "polyvagal theory," and in less than an hour, I learned more than I could have imagined about breathing. In fact, in all my years of breathing in and out, and in coaching people to "calm down" and "take a deep breath" to decrease their stress, I never truly understood how much breathing alone affects our physical and mental health, at the most basic neurochemical level. Let me explain.

According to Rebecca Knowles (2022), as we breathe in deeply, we relax the large muscles of the diaphragm, which when held tight "squeeze" on the primary nerves running between our brain and stomach. Because these nerves regulate both the sympathetic and parasympathetic nervous systems, when the diaphragm is held tight, these nerves receive signals from the muscles of the diaphragm to send forth messenger chemicals to turn on the stress response and prepare us for survival in life-threatening situations. When relaxed, the opposite system engages. In turn, these change the way we think, function, and react, and as we move into adrenal activation by holding our breath tight, our fight-flight-freeze responses are primed to react. These neurochemicals then fuel how we think and feel, and they create an emotional response to perceived threat.

NATUROPATHIC WISDOM

Let me explain this in simpler terms. In a stress response, let's say being startled by someone coming up silently behind us in a dark alley, we instinctively take in a fast, sharp breath that immediately tightens the muscles of the diaphragm and puts pressure on the large nerves that activate both what we are aware of, such as our thoughts and emotions, and the body's responses for things like heart rate and blood pressure. So, simply put, that sharp intake of breath activates a complex series of neurochemical responses which prepare our bodies for danger. When this happens, the body responds to these "stress signals" in many ways, with the most obvious of these reactions including faster and more shallow breaths, an increase in heart rate, an increase in the production of stomach acid to empty out the stomach, and movement of blood towards our hands and feet for improved defenses and reaction speed. But as these changes in our bodies occur, the mind also responds by increasing our sensory awareness, hyper-focusing to prepare for threat, and with the protective feelings of fear and/or aggression.

But now that our body systems are prepared for defense, let's assume that the perceived predator doesn't come, and this pressure that is being held tightly within our diaphragm is carried over for a long period of time; when this occurs, we keep using these stress-reactive breathing patterns. What is the result? Yes, you guessed it, repeated neurochemical signaling, deep within the body, which keeps us primed for survival from immediate threat. But in so doing, the energy required to sustain this priming also places the long-term sustainability and wellness of the individual on hold. Emotionally, the individual has heightened sensitivity, feels too ramped up to concentrate, and both anxiety and eventually depression (as the neurochemical correction to long-standing anxiety) are the result. In this way, the individual who holds their breath becomes out-of-sync for relaxed, healthful, sustainable living.

Thus, truly, the way that we breathe, how relaxed our diaphragm is when we breathe, the quality of the air that comes into our lungs when breathing, and even the literal amount of oxygen we take in when we breathe essentially regulates our entire nervous system. This means that large, full, deep breaths, where the diaphragm expands to decrease pressure on our sympathetic and parasympathetic nerves, rid our bodies of unhealthy stress responses.

Breathing and Airborne Chemical Sensitivities

During the height of my illness, I could not breathe well. I was diagnosed with asthma, and I had also become so extremely sensitive to certain fragrances and chemicals in the air that these would cause me to go into immediate anaphylactic shock when I encountered them. As expected, my anxiety was also at an all-time high when these sensitivities were at their worst. To this day, I still use a service dog who is trained to identify various allergens and alert me to these in my surroundings before I need to use an epinephrine pen.

But since his training, because my dog also regularly goes everywhere with me, I have noticed that he can also accurately detect stress signals in the people around me. Armed with this information, I've begun talking about airborne chemicals and fragrance-activated stress responses with my clients, and remarkably I've discovered that most of the kids I see are also triggered with headaches and 'fuzzy thinking' by reactions to a variety of fragrances and cleaning products in their various home and school environments. Within these discussions, a few trends have emerged. It seems that commercial air fresheners, laundry products, a variety of professional cleaning agents, and several perfumes are the most problematic.

While I had never checked the literature before authoring this book for the topic of fragrance and symptomology, when I did, I was not surprised to learn that my observations about fragrances were confirmed in several large studies. In the most comprehensive of these, Steinemann (2016) reports that "fragranced products have been associated with a range of adverse health effects, such as migraine headaches, asthma attacks, respiratory difficulties, neurological problems, mucosal symptoms, and contact dermatitis." Steinemann adds that in the U.S., 19% of the entire population reports breathing difficulties, headaches, fogginess in thinking, and other health problems when exposed to air fresheners and deodorizers, with 10.9% of all people reporting physical health problems from the scent of certain laundry products.

With fragrance sensitivity that can result in headaches, sinus pain, foggy thinking, and a few of the more classical allergic reactions reported in so many of the kids in my practice, it seems obvious to me that if a fragrance can cause someone to suffer from a headache within only a few minutes of exposure, long-term exposure to these fragrances will obviously have a negative effect on feelings of wellness and on one's overall ability to think, learn, and react. Why then are we not looking more carefully at these, especially in schools and other settings where kids have long-term exposure? What if environmental chemicals and fragrances are changing the ways that kids breathe?

Today, I now listen very carefully when a child tells me that a certain smell makes them feel ill, because these scents and chemicals need to be eliminated whenever possible. For some kids, this means that a change in cleaning products, air fresheners, or perfumes using more nature-based products is necessary. Last, I am reminded here that there is simply no substitute for clean, fresh, outdoor air, especially when this can be obtained from nature. For this reason, I also recommend frequent walks in nature, and when that is not possible, I promote opening windows (especially after it has rained) to clear indoor, polluted airspaces.

NATUROPATHIC WISDOM

Breath Work and Teaching Kids to Breathe

In my practice, like many mental health practitioners, I have a couch. But instead of using it for counseling, I use it to teach children and teens how to breathe. While they are lying down, I ask them to put their hands directly over their diaphragm to see if there is any rise or fall occurring there. When we start, most have only minimal rise and fall, and as they work to force a rise and fall in their diaphragm, the breath pattern becomes "wobbly" looking, from both side-to-side and top-to-bottom. From there, I specifically tell kids what I am looking for in their breathing (a full, stable rise and fall in the diaphragm), and I ask them to open their mouths, the width of two fingers, then breathe in through their mouths, taking in as much air as they can force into their lungs. In this breathing exercise, the out breath is done through the nose. I usually have kids do this for at least ten big breaths, while continuing to check for an even pattern of rise and fall across the diaphragm.

Once they practice this a few times, most of them start yawning. From there, I encourage them to yawn 'as big as they can,' and 'whenever they feel the need to.' I then continue to coach them in taking in as much air as they can physically hold, filling up their entire lungs 'like two barrels.' I repeat this for one hundred breaths. When teaching young children, or those who cannot get through the breathing practices above, I encourage big breathing by having them take big breaths to then blow that air through a straw to make bubbles. For older kids, while I am teaching them how to breathe, I am also giving them information about the neurology behind using their breath to control their thoughts and emotions.

By the time kids do this breathing exercise for one hundred breaths, many will be relaxed enough to want to sleep. In fact, I will sometimes even bet kids who cannot sleep at night that I can help them go to sleep right here in my office. I usually win these bets, and when parents come to pick up their sleepy child, I explain that we simply have turned off the pressure on their 'big nerves,' which both calm them down and help them relax.

In my experience, I have found that once children learn to control their breathing and understand why it is important, they have learned one of the first and most important tools I can give them for controlling their stress responses, their attention, their anxiety, and their impulsive reactions. Simply put, full, relaxed breathing is the best medicine for eliminating stress.

Additional recommendations that I often share to address breathing and the stress responses in my clients include singing lessons (these generally teach breath control) and formal breath therapy through programs like those offered at Unyte Health Online. For kids who cannot learn to use their breath well on their own, I refer them for biofeedback training, breath coaching, or work with a licensed breath therapist. With tight and arrested breathing being the quickest path to an undue stress response, it is well worth the time for parents and educators to monitor, facilitate, and formally teach good breathing patterns to all children.

CHAPTER 11

The Need for Restful Sleep

Chapter 11

It also is obvious that we all need adequate, restful sleep. But for today's kids, especially teenagers, late-night homework, limited physical exercise, and unresolved daytime stressors have dramatically decreased sleep quality (Phillips, Johnson, Shirey, and Rice, 2020). Added to this, many of today's youth keep their electronic devices next to their beds (Fuller, Lehman, Hicks, & Novick, 2017) and when being honest, of those who sleep with these devices, high numbers of today's youth report texting, talking, video chats, and staying connected with peers on and off throughout the night. According to the World Health Organization, many of today's children also struggle with video-game addiction, with 8.4 percent of all children worldwide losing significant sleep due to video game play. With all these disruptions to children's sleep, and when combined with the numerous factors that cause light pollution and melatonin disruption mentioned in the above chapters, is it any wonder that kids are not receiving the beneficial recovery from sleep that is needed for healthful living?

NATUROPATHIC WISDOM

The Effects of Lost Sleep in Children and Teens

According to Boksem, Meijmam, and Lorist (2005), once children become cognitively tired (irrespective of how much physical energy they still have available), their day-time attention decreases significantly. Irregular and/or less than optimal sleep also results in a decrease in one's ability to perform tasks of accurate sensory processing (Rajaei et al., 2020). This means that poor sleep increases sensory sensitivity and disrupts the physiological state of mind and body neuromodulation, which has been shown to increase learning, attention, and mental health disorders in children according to Smaldone, Honig, and Byrne (2007).

In studies specifically looking at anxiety and arousal for their relationship to sleep, Pitvik, Joncas, and Busby (1999) found that sleep spindles (which are markers for deep and restful sleep) significantly decrease when children sleep in heightened states of anxiety or arousal. Furthermore, researchers have also concluded that highly stressed children engage in more sleep talking, teeth grinding, and disruptive snoring at night.

In their examination of screen-time before bed, Li et al. (2007) found that the use of a computer before bed negatively affected sleep and increased children's levels of daytime anxiety. But what about getting that homework done? Interestingly, Curcio, Ferrara, and De Gennaro, in their 2006 study found that adequate sleep had a more positive impact on grades than did time spent on homework. Owens and Kaplan (2005) also examined the sleep patterns of over 3,000 children in the U.S., China, and England, and their study found that children who had more homework and other daytime stress demands had more difficulty falling asleep and staying asleep at night. This study further concluded that children living in the U.S. and China (countries where more homework is assigned) are less attentive and more anxious during the day than their counterparts in other parts of the world.

In one last study on sleep and school performance, in a longitudinal review of school start times, Wahistrom (2000) found that students who started the school day even one hour later were more likely to be alert, present, and focused, with significantly fewer reports of anxiety and depresssion. With these findings, it becomes clear that children need proper rest. Adequate sleep also appears to improve sensory processing, regulate stress responses, and decrease the propensity for learning, mental health, and behavior disorders.

Case Study, the Boy Who Didn't Sleep

On my client intake questionnaire, which every new family completes, I specifically ask those entering my practice about daytime sensory sensitivities, sleeping habits, nighttime waking, night terrors, and the actual amount of time that kids are sleeping. I also ask how hot or cold a child feels when sleeping (in my experience hot sleepers tend to have more learning disabilites). Last, I ask about bed-wetting, as this too seems to correlate with learning and mental health disorders for many children.

Several years ago, using this questionnaire, I tested a young boy who simply wasn't sleeping. He had always been a poor sleeper, woke many times during the night, was still wetting his bed at the age of seven, and as a second-grade student, had been diagnosed with both ADHD and dyslexia. He also struggled with anxiety and reported not feeling well, with frequent migraine headaches and stom-achaches, although physical causes for these had been ruled out. When he did sleep for short periods of time, he slept 'hot' and sweated to the point that his clothes and bedding were soaked through by waking. Socially he was quick to react, impulsive, and very aggressive. On rare occasions when asked to play with peers, he turned down play dates claiming that he was just too tired to play. By day's end he was fidgety, restless, and often explosive, with full-blown tantrums and meltdowns that lasted as long as one hour frequently occuring before bed.

Although initially reluctant, due to the fact that her son didn't ever seem tired or sleepy, at my recommendation the family sought a sleep study at one of the local children's hospitals and discovered that he was waking approximatley forty-two times per hour. Using a child-sized continuous

Chapter 11

positive airway pressure (CPAP) machine, this boy came to me two years later for reassessment. Not only had his attention and behavior challenges resolved, in testing he had also increased his IQ by thirty-two points, was reading at grade level, and had several close friends that were regular playmates. Most notably, though, this boy looked like a different kid. I've thought a lot about him since, and I've wondered what would have happened had this family treated their son with a stimulant medication, as was prescribed for his impulsive and inattentive behaviors. How long would it have been before he was properly treated for his sleep disorder. How many other kids diagnosed with these same mental health conditions are suffering from sleep disorders?

Recommendations to Improve Sleep

This brings me to the following conclusions. Children need to sleep. In addition to addressing light and noise pollution in sleeping quarters, it seems clear to me that parents must regulate electronic devices and games when these interfere with sleep. Schools also need to have productive conversations about how much homework is too much and adjust accordingly when school work cuts into sleeping time. Doctors, mental health workers, and teachers should also pay more attention to reports about children who are not sleeping and refer these for sleep studies. It also seems prudent that when kids are 'hot sleepers,' the possibility for abnormalities in sleep should be ruled out before other diagnoses and treatments are implemented.

For teens, I've recommmended sleep tracking devices to monitor sleep abnormalities, especially when the causes for poor sleep are not clear or there is no 'buy in' from the teen about their need for sleep. I also regularly recommend the implementation of nighttime breathing exercises and other meditative practices, along with relaxing bedtime routines to calm the minds of children who are going to bed in states of stress or over-arousal. When evening tantrums are common, I start looking for ways to shorten the child's school day to prevent children from resorting to stress-reactive melt-down behaviors that are caused by an energy shortage or a too-long school day.

CHAPTER 12

Forest Bathing

Chapter 12

According to Li (2018, p. 3) "we have never been so divorced from nature." Based on the findings of one study conducted by the Environmental Protection Agency (2022), the average American spends 93 percent of his or her time indoors. From an evolutionary perspective then, with humans living outdoors and/or in close proximity to nature for most of our existence, what are the impacts of disconnection from the natural world?

The Research on Shinrin-Yoku

A few months ago, I had the unique pleasure of interviewing the highly respected Dr. Yoshifumi Miyazaki (2022), on behalf of the US Autism Association. Dr. Miyazaki is known the world over for his clinical research on the physiological effects of *Shinrin-yoku* or Forest Bathing. In this interview Dr. Miyazaki shared findings from multiple field studies in which randomized clinical trials, which are the gold standard in allopathic medicine, compared various health markers for those who regularly spent time in nature and those who only spent time in the city. The findings of his research were quite eye-opening.

While we all know that spending time in nature makes us feel good, Dr. Miyazaki's research tells us why. Across twenty-four different studies, researchers found that *Nature Bathing*, in as few as fifteen-minute increments at a time, "lowered concentrations of cortisol [which is necessary for proper functioning of the immune system], lowered pulse rates, lowered both systolic and diastolic blood pressure, increased parasympathetic nerve activity [which calms the central nervous system], lowered sympathetic nerve activity [which reacts with a number of body changes when stress is high], and decreased blood glucose." Within these studies, Dr. Miyazaki and his research team also found that time spent in nature relieves psychological tension, depression, anger, fatigue, and even mental confusion while enhancing human vigor.

In an additional study conducted in 2017 at the Nippon Medical School researchers found that spending only three days in nature significantly boosted Natural Killer (NK) cells, which are critical for their action on intracellular anti-cancer proteins. Additional findings on the benefits of spending time in nature, according to Dr. Miyazaki, also strongly support the conclusion that the forest is simply a good restorative environment for human beings for many reasons that are not yet fully understood.

After I completed the interview and when we were no longer on camera, I asked Dr. Miyazaki why he thought that Forest Bathing was proving to be such a powerful tool in treating so many different conditions. Off-record, he told me that there were too many variables to consider in isolation but that anyone who wants to live a healthy life must spend at least thirty minutes per day, outdoors, in filtered sun, and in close proximity to trees (the older the better). He added that walks among nature's plants seem to help us acquire some sort of 'necessary healing properties' that are abundantly present in the forest but are nonexistent in other environments. As we discussed this further, he added that we "still know so very little about how plants and trees interact with each other, at a cellular level, and with our own human bodies, but the more we learn, the more amazing the findings become."

Naturopathic Views on Spending Time in Nature

While the study of Forest Bathing is a relatively new phenomenon, naturopaths from around the globe have been touting the benefits of spending time outside for centuries. With the benefits ranging from clean, fresh air and filtered sunshine, to relaxing walks and deep breaths of the various natural chemicals that are emitted by living trees and plants, the naturopath considers time in nature to be one of most restorative practices in any healing tradition. For many naturopaths, even the magnetic vibrations between the earth, the plants and trees, and the human body are believed to have healing properties.

NATUROPATHIC WISDOM

So, with new studies in allopathic medicine now also establishing the benefits of spending time in nature, within the same scientifically rigorous studies that are employed in testing new pharmaceutical drug treatments, perhaps at least in this area, the naturopath and allopath are no longer as divided as they have historically been in the past.

As proposed by Christine Meier (2022) when engaging in nature bathing, the following recommendations should guide you.

> First, find a spot. Make sure you have left your phone and camera behind. You are going to be walking aimlessly and slowly. You don't need any devices. Let your body be your guide. Listen to where it wants to take you. Follow your nose. And take your time. It doesn't matter if you don't get anywhere. You are not going anywhere. You are savoring the sounds, smells, and sights of nature and letting the forest in. Listen to the birds singing and the breeze rustling in the leaves of the trees. Look at the different greens of the trees and the sunlight filtering through the branches. Smell the fragrance of the forest and breathe in the natural aromatherapy of phytoncides. Taste the freshness of the air as you take deep breaths. Place your hands on the trunk of a tree. Dip your fingers or toes in a stream. Lie on the

Chapter 12

ground. Drink in the flavor of the forest and release your sense of joy and calm. This is your sixth sense, a state of mind. Now you have connected with nature, you have crossed the bridge to happiness.

I believe that for most children and teens, the benefits of time in nature are enhanced even further because of their developing sensory processing systems. As I have watched my own children and the children of others across many diverse settings in modern life, I have arrived at the conclusion that there is no time more precious for the developing child than the time spent freely exploring and playfully interacting with the bounties of nature. This leads me to my favorite topic in all of naturopathy, the study of botanicals within aromatherapy and herbology.

CHAPTER 13

The Healing Properties of Plants

Chapter 13

For about ten years, in addition to running my private practice, I also owned and operated a private special needs school that served approximately 175 children with severe learning, behavior, and mental health disorders. In my school, one of the primary goals was to get kids off their medications, as much as was possible. To do this we had to find a variety of alternative ways to deal with difficult behaviors while also teaching these children academics. We had many successes at my school, and we also had some failures. But for anyone who attended, one of the most memorable things that I consider successful was the daily use of organic aromatherapy oils to help the children calm when calming was needed, and to assist them with focusing and alerting when their energy was too low to focus and attend. For me personally this meant that I washed and dried approximately 150 aromatherapy scented wash rags at the end of every school day. For a full decade after the school closed, I still smelled both citrus and lavender every time I turned on my dryer.

NATUROPATHIC WISDOM

The Chemistry of Essential Oils

In what has become one of my favorite books on my bookshelf, Dr. David Stewart, in his book the *Chemistry of Essential Oils Made Simple: God's Love Manifest in Molecules*, defines essential oils as the "the volatile lipid (oil) portion of the fluids of a plant" (2016, p. 51). As a chemist himself, Stewart adds that across the plant kingdom, there are approximately 400,000 known plants, and each contains several hundred different 'phenolic compounds,' or 'essences'; Stewart adds that at the time he wrote his book, no plant yet had ever been fully analyzed in a laboratory to include all its underlying trace compounds. This means that the possible combinations of phenolic compounds or essences available from the vast array of plants on the earth constitute a truly staggering number.

But why do plants contain so many different phenolic compounds? In short, these compounds help the plant defend and propagate. Phenolic compounds or essences function as the plant's immune system. In addition to attracting substances that increase the plant's chances for pollination, these also provide color or camouflage, sun attraction or sun blocking properties, defend against herbivores, give the plant antibacterial and antifungal activities, and allow the plant to repair, heal, and restore itself when injured or diseased (Mandal, Chakraborty, & Dey, 2010).

Chapter 13

Why Essential Oils are Beneficial to Humans

With so many known properties relating to how plants protect themselves, we are only now beginning to uncover the vast number of benefits that these various plant essence molecules could have on human health and wellness. What is clear, however, is this: when properly extracted and administered, using only high quality, therapeutic grade oils, at least some of the benefits from these plant essence chemicals are shared with humans (Lin et al. in 2106).

In an extensive review of the literature across large numbers of published studies focusing on the benefits of essential oils in healing, Babar et al. (2015) found that aroma molecules in plants are 'very potent chemicals.' In their review, researchers report that essential plant oils can: effectively rid the environment of diseases with antibacterial, antiviral, and antifungal origins; have anti-inflammatory, immune boosting, and hormonal regulation properties; act favorably on glandular and circulatory responses; and alter cognitive processes to increase memory, improve calmness, and boost alertness and attention. Babar (2015) adds that because of the way these chemicals work in the body to resemble actual hormones, they also cause the brain to release large numbers of 'neuro messengers' such as serotonin, endorphin, noradrenalin, and epinephrine, which normalize and regulate the nervous system as well as other body systems. The review concludes to state that the use of essential oils, when administered therapeutically, can provide relief from numerous physical and mental health ailments.

The Importance of High Quality, Therapeutic Grade Oils

To control costs, many essential oil products sold today, however, include fillers that contain alcohols, chemical dilutants, and less expensive oil substitutes. In addition, because of the amount of plant matter that is needed to produce even a single ounce of essential plant oil, any pesticides, herbicides, fungicides, or other unhealthy chemicals used to grow that plant, along with chemicals present in the soil, have the potential to be heavily concentrated in the resulting oil. So do not be fooled by labels! Oils claiming to be 100% natural or 100% pure can still contain elevated levels of toxic chemicals.

Therefore, when purchasing oils, especially for use with children, parents should focus on acquiring essential oils only under the label **100% Pure Essential Oil of High, Therapeutic Grade**. However, even under this label, because no U.S. government agency formally 'grades' oils, some additional research on the source of the oil being used is often necessary to ensure that the oil is properly sourced for safety. When purchasing oils, I usually recommend that the oil be sourced from its natural habitat, whenever possible, or sourced from a certified organic farm. I also want to know if any other ingredients are included in the oil. Last, I recommend that parents test oils by placing a small amount of the oil on the fingers. When there is an oily residue present, I have found that the oil is unlikely to be that of a pure essential oil; true essential oils are rarely greasy. While finding high-quality oils is not always easy, there are several reputable companies producing high-grade therapeutic essential oils, and these usually employ strict quality controls with independent, third-party verifications. So once again, before you consider essential oils, you need to do your research.

The Safety of Essential Oils for Children

When using essential oils with children, I also refer specifically to a safety report published by the Children's Hospital of Philadelphia for additional guidelines. In their 2020 report, the authors specifically recommend the following: 1) children under the age of three should not be considered for aromatherapy treatments; 2) lavender, peppermint, ginger, and citrus (such as sweet orange or mandarin), are well researched for their safety with children; 3) essential oils should only be purchased from a reliable source; 4) never let a child put aromatherapy oils into their mouths; even diluted oils can be harmful when swallowed; 5) never apply pure essential oils directly to a child's skin; 6) never use heat to diffuse an oil's fragrance into the air as essential oils are flammable; and 7) the use of camphor, clove, eucalyptus, thyme, tea tree, and wintergreen oils should be used with caution in young children unless these are recommended under the direct advisement and care of a licensed naturopathic or qualified allopathic physician.

Plant-Based Medicines and Psychopharmacology

With so many potential chemical combinations possible in plants, and data that is still in its infancy for documenting the potential healing properties that are possible through aromatherapy, you might find it surprising to know that almost all medicines in use today, within the entire field of pharmacology, have their origins in the botanical sciences. According to Harvard University (2011), throughout history, human medicines are frequently based on plant-derived compounds. But in the past century, as science advanced, and the chemical properties of plants were able to be seen and studied under increasingly powerful microscopes, chemists learned to extract the active ingredients from these natural sources and reproduce them in the laboratory with slight chemical changes.

Chapter 13

Thus, by studying the various chemicals that were found within the well-documented healing properties of plants, and building on these to establish a growing body of chemical research, by the 1960s, chemists had formally begun to create their own unique chemical composition 'drugs,' to replicate some of the medicinal properties that had been observed in botanical medicine for centuries (Katiyar, Gupta, Kanjilal, & Katiyar, 2012). For most naturopaths, this is where the problem with many of the pharmacological and psychopharmacological treatments began.

Simply put, the naturopath would suggest that once the medicinal properties of various plants were extracted and delivered in isolation, away from the hundreds of other lessor chemical compounds present in the original plant, or the chemical composition was altered, something important was lost in the medicine. Added to this, and because researchers cannot simply patent a chemical composition that already exists in nature, changes in the molecular structures of these natural plant extract chemicals were made. While these are not deemed to be that problematic within allopathic medicine, the naturopathic practitioner would wholeheartedly disagree.

In fact, the naturopath takes the position that while changes to the molecular structure of most of the chemical compounds that are found in plants can effectively mimic the medicinal or treatment property of the original plant from which the medicine was derived, these small changes become very important to stasis and the overall performance of the medicine on the body. It is also believed that within these extractions and modifications, medication side-effects, which were not necessarily present within use of the whole original plant emerged (Stewart, 2016).

I understand that this position will continue to be heavily criticized. Modern allopathic medicine is a true miracle in so many ways. But in my mind, it makes sense that as we eradicate the very 'nature-based perfection' that was present in the original healing plants of the earth and attempt to replicate and reproduce these healing properties with chemical substitutes, we should at least be asking if we are forever altering the true, holistic, healing properties of the plants of the earth from which original medicine was derived. Furthermore, because the process for creating medicine is the same across all industries for both prescription drugs and for over-the-counter medicines, vitamins, and supplements, are these too less beneficial than the original plants? Finally, as so many of our healing plants are becoming extinct, are we losing the deep healing properties of the plants of the earth? As we consider these questions, I think we should at least do whatever is necessary to preserve as many whole-plant species as is possible until we know more. I also believe that we may still discover that all parts of a medicinal plant, not just the most prominent, are beneficial to healing processes. Researchers Rasoanaivo, Wright, Willcox, and Gilbert (2011) have specifically focused on using whole plant extracts versus single compounds for the treatment of malaria and their findings on the synergy and positive interactions between the primary and secondary plant components are quite remarkable.

Whole Herbs as Medicine

Because I personally believe in the synergy of the hundreds of chemical components present in healing plants, when possible, I recommend and support the use of natural, whole, plant-based herbs, delivered in the form of fresh or dried harvested roots, leaves, and flowers, when these are available. Many plants are medicine and should be used only under the direction of a trained naturopathic doctor or herbologist. It is also helpful to understand why the field of pharmacology doesn't investigate whole, plant-based cures: simply put, creating and delivering a new drug is expensive. So, because whole plants cannot be owned exclusively, there is very little incentive for the field of pharmacology to use plants in their natural form. Thus, access to plant-based medicine is quite difficult to obtain.

When I completed my naturopathic studies, I specifically chose to focus more in-depth on coursework in herbology. As I studied this topic, I also collected a personal-use apothecary containing over seventy raw medicinal plants (either chopped whole or ground parts). As I learned, I also began to use these to build my own health. But even with course-work in both pharmacology and herbology, where I live, I cannot legally recommend or use herbs in my practice. That said, I believe I can still share some basic recommendations for the use of herbs, drawn from those practitioners who are licensed, for parents who want to explore herbology when treating their children.

Recommendations for Using Herbs with Children

First off, herbal plants, taken in medicinal doses, must be treated as real medicine. As such, these should not be used carelessly or without the support of a trained (and in my state licensed) herbologist or naturopathic doctor. Next, the trace amounts of plant material present in most herbal teas or over-the-counter supplements are approved for their safety with children, but parents should still be careful and read warning labels on these products. It might also be helpful to know that most herbal supplements are simply extracts taken from the primary medicinal properties of the original plant, so in most cases, these too do not contain the entire chemical composition of the original healing plant. In addition, as is true for the quality of essential oils used in aromatherapy, all serious use of herbs as medicine should be drawn from clean, natural, and/or certified organically grown sources. Beyond these basic and woefully limited recommendations, I will add this—in herbology, perhaps more than in any of the other various practices of naturopathy, the burden of careful and cautious research falls squarely on the shoulders of parents. I have personally been working through various herbology training courses for well over a decade now and I will say that even now, I still feel extremely naïve in my own knowledge about this vast field of study. So, as an additional caution, I will add that in this area, parents should not try to go it alone. In using medicinal levels of herbs with children, I recommend that you consult with an herbal medicine expert who is both qualified and legally able to help you.

Even though the use of herbs for children can be quite difficult, for those who have taken the time and effort to learn about and find skilled herbalists to help, the benefits that I have seen, while usually much slower than those obtained through modern psychopharmacological approaches, can be quite remarkable. I have seen successful treatment for ADHD, depression, anxiety, traumatic brain injury, and even mood and thought disorders using only herbal treatments. I personally also attribute much of my own healing and wellness success to the careful and practiced use of herbs as medicine.

NATUROPATHIC WISDOM

Medical Cannabinoid

As another topic of interest under this category, I can also personally and professionally attest to the benefits of cannabinoid oil, especially when applied trans-dermally directly to the brain stem under a doctor's care. In attempts to understand why the various molecular components within the marijuana plant finally cured my seizure disorders, while also successfully treating nerve pain that had required years-long use of prescription pain medicine, I set out to find an expert.

In so doing, I discovered and connected with a leading neuropsychiatrist in Florida who specializes in using real-time, EEG imaging data to select and administer specific CBD and CBD/THC blends for use under license and prescription in the treatment of various physical and neuropsychiatric conditions. With a body of research that is highly regarded by both allopathic and naturopathic doctors alike, I also started referring some of my more challenging clients to Dr. Ron Aung-Din.

Since we met, he has helped about thirty of my clients by providing an alternative and effective path for necessary treatments in psychiatry, conditions that would have otherwise required psychiatric medication. Because Dr. Aung-Din's work is well-documented, I will not try to repeat its premise here. But he is a true pioneer in this field. An official interview with him on this topic is available to the public on the US Autism Association's YouTube channel and within the US Autism Association's Video Streaming Library (2022).

Considering Homeopathy?

While not specifically drawing only from botanicals, the field of homeopathy may also have some interesting merits for its use of plant-, animal-, and mineral-based chemical compounds for use in the treatment of illness and disease. Thus, for parents who would like to explore this field, which is included under the umbrella of naturopathy, I will provide a basic description about what homeopathy entails, along with a few things to consider when using homeopathy with children.

Homeopathy's History and Principles

The field of homeopathy originated in the early 1800s, under the work of German physician Samuel Fredrick Hahnemann. Disillusioned with medical practices of his day, Hahnemann believed that under *God Given Law*, the body could recognize certain substances drawn from either the 'vegetable, animal, or mineral kingdom,' and use these to heal itself.

NATUROPATHIC WISDOM

According to Panos and Heimlich (1980), and as drawn from their book *Homeopathic Medicine at Home*, in home-opathy, there are three laws that lay the foundation for the healing principles of this method. In the first of these, the *Law of Similars*, homeopaths believed that 'like is cured by like.' What this means is this: when a healthy person takes certain substances, and this results in symptoms that are the same as the symptoms associated with some disease or medical condition, then that substance can be used to effec-tively treat that disease or condition. So which substances are used? These are determined within the second law, which is referred to as the *Law of Proving*, where healthy people, using a double-blind method (some get the substance while others get a placebo) are given daily doses of various sub-stances and their symptoms are carefully recorded. In this way, several hundred substances have been evaluated and are now included within the homeopathic pharmacy. Finally, within the third law, which is called the *Law of Potentization*, the substances are prepared for use. Here's where things get interesting. In homeopathy, the Law of Potentization states that *higher rates of dilution provide more potency*. Yes, you read that correctly. What this means is that in each preparation, where a substance is diluted and shaken (referred to as suc-cussion), the process itself gives strength and healing powers to the remedy. With dilutions rates that range from 200 to 100,000 (at 100,000 the substance has been homeopathically diluted 100,000 times, with a dilution rate of one part per

Chapter 13

100 parts) homeopaths agree that at the highest (and most potent) levels, the resulting remedy might in fact no longer contain any actual molecules from the original substance (Panos & Heimlich, 1980).

For this reason, homeopathy is one of the most controversial practices included under the naturopathic umbrella. But despite its basic principles (especially for those relating to potency) and within logic that doesn't necessarily make sense to most people, six million people report using one or more homeopathic remedies in the U.S. each year (Dossett, M. L., & Yeh, 2018). In another large population study performed by researchers Relton, Cooper, Viksveen, Fibert, and Thomas (2017), it is reported that 3 percent of all children in the U.S. take daily homeopathic remedies.

My Views and Recommendations on Homeopathy

As another area of naturopathy in which I regularly give my referred clients a quick 'heads up,' I have had dozens of families report back to me that while they were initially skeptical, they now believe that homeopathic remedies gave their children much-needed health improvements. So, I cannot tell you if or why homeopathy works. As a general recommendation I guess I would not suggest taking out a loan to pay for homeopathic services.

But also, as the ex-wife of a theoretical, particle physicist, I can say that even in hard science, we now understand (though we don't know why) that within the basic components of all molecular structures, when broken down into their smallest subatomic particles, some pretty strange things happen when we observe and interact with these particles. In fact, if you want to be truly mind-blown spend a day or two reading about particle and quantum physics. So, while I personally am still a bit skeptical about homeopathy, I leave open the possibility that while not yet well explained or understood in medicine, science might one day find medical merit in the practices of homeopathy, due to the very way in which homeopathic remedies are prepared. In the meantime, I will add this: we can at least say that homeopathy is safe and that the practice will 'do no harm.'

My Homeopathy Story

In closing I will share a personal homeopathy story. During my final year of severe illness, and after I had started searching for alternative medical treatments late in my illness, I met with a licensed homeopathic physician. Based on his recommendation, I tried a three-part combination of homeopathic medicines (I do not now recall what was in them). But by taking these diligently every four hours, across a two-day cycle, which also included drinking lots of water, I did get a welcome five-day reprieve from my hives. At the time this was incredibly significant to me, as I had not gone a single day in over two years without having hives on at least 50 percent of my body. That said, I could never replicate the results, using the same remedies, and I even tried just drinking similar amounts of water, but the results never came again. With such a remarkable moment in my own healing journey, and one that still stands out prominently in my memory, I will certainly never discredit the practices of homeopathy for my own lack of understanding.

CHAPTER 14

Bathing & Water Therapies

Chapter 14

According to Gianfaldoni et al. (2017), as reported in their extensive review on the history of baths and thermal treatments in medicine, the benefits of hydrotherapy (water therapy) and thermal cures (sitting in or using water at various temperatures) have been well-documented throughout history. Beginning in ancient times and carrying forward to this day, man has always recognized the beneficial properties of water and has enjoyed bathing in and using water at various temperatures for healing.

Hydrotherapy Through the Ages

In fact, within numerous cultures, clean, pure water is even revered as 'sacred.' Briar (2019) shares that as far back as ancient Egypt, the life-giving force of water was believed to underlie all of creation. In the days of the great pharaohs, water became 'a spirit god' with the ability to 'birth and heal' all living things. Moving forward in history, the ancient Greeks first recorded the medical benefits of bathing, with their earliest written accounts of water therapy depicting the healing properties of bathing in sulfur-rich springs to heal skin diseases and alleviate joint and muscular pain (Tsitsis, et al. 2013). Hippocrates and Plato also both wrote extensively about the restorative nature of 'thermal waters' and described the benefits of soaking in these for the treatment of disease; Hippocrates even accurately described the effects of hot and cold baths on the human body (Gianfaldoni et al., 2017).

Drawing from early beliefs about the healing properties of water, the rise, fall, and rise again of bathing in mineral springs, bath houses, and public bathing centers, eventually under the more medical sounding term of 'thermalism' eventually evolved, with both hot and cold baths believed to successfully treat everything from fatigue and stress to more serious injuries, such as those of the wounded military soldier or the terminally ill (Michaelides, 2014). By the 1800s, with a long-standing history of healing, biochemical scientists formally began to analyze natural hot springs and thermal water sources for their chemical constitutions. When this occurred, the fields of 'hydrotherapy' (immersion of the body in heated or cooled water for therapeutic purposes) and 'balneotherapy' (cures obtained through soaking in naturally occurring mineral-rich springs) officially became reputable forms of treatment in the medical sciences. For a time, doctors of the day were even convinced that for each disease there was an appropriate medicinal spring somewhere on earth to treat it (Jackson, 1990).

In the years that have followed, both balneotherapy and hydrotherapy were used extensively within the medical establishment, with favorable outcomes. But these practices

Chapter 14

were also misused. In treating those with mental health conditions in particular, the practice of submersion or spraying with water at near-freezing temperatures was one of the more abusive water-therapy practices. With the use of ice and heat packs now taking over for most of the water-based therapy of the past in the field of allopathic medicine, the fields of balneotherapy and hydrotherapy have seen a tremendous increase in the field of tourism, especially as these have been combined with other treatments in naturopathy, such as the use of herbal baths, mud packs, relaxing exercise, and massage therapy. Today, the water-based therapies of the past are mostly present in our modern-day spas, resorts, and beach-front vacations. But, according to van Tubergen and van der Linden (2002), as has been true throughout history, the practices of 'restorative tourism' where people flock to ocean-side resorts, naturally occurring springs, and various other water-featured vacations continue to feed the soul and restore the body in much the same way as it did for our ancestors throughout history. But with so much recorded history on the potential healing properties of water and water-based therapies, what does the research have to say?

NATUROPATHIC WISDOM

Clinical Studies on the Benefits of Hydrotherapy

In clinical studies, hydrotherapy has been heavily researched and clearly documented for its usefulness for the successful treatment of a variety of musculoskeletal conditions. In fact, it is still considered to be the primary 'standard of care' for most medical treatments in the field of neuro-muscular rehabilitation (Barker, et al., 2014).

In children, various studies show that the benefits of bathing, swimming, and soaking in naturally occurring waters and mineral springs include: improved motor performance, the balancing of sensory processing systems and increased tolerance for sensory stimuli, increases in active range of motion and movement, improved postural stability, relaxation of spastic muscles, improved circulation, and even increases in language development according to a systematic review of the literature conducted by Getz, Hutzler, and Vermeer (2006).

For children with special needs, research reports suggest significant improvements in muscular strength and endurance along with improved motor coordination (Yilmaz, Yanardag, Birkan, & Bumin, 2004). For those with autism and other developmental disorders, Mortimer, and Kumar (2014) found decreases in stereotypical movements, hyperactive behavior, and anxiety along with significant improvements in self-confidence, social performance, and relationship-building skills.

Chapter 14

Across all populations, various water-based therapies have also been proven to create physiological changes that contribute to vasodilation, increased blood flow, reduction of arterial stiffness, improved vascular function, cellular oxygenation, and decreased sleep-related stress (Jiyeon, Lee, & Yi, 2019). In one study, researchers Wilcock, Cronin, and Hing (2006) even demonstrated that the simple act of sitting in a warm body of water was so effective at healing, that physiological changes similar to those seen within thirty minutes of cardiovascular exercise were observed; these changes included the improvement of cardiovascular function, increased cardiac output, decreased atherosclerotic plaque formations, decreased vascular resistance, increased organ function, improved insulin-sensitivity, increased oxygen carrying capacity in the cells, and improved plasma lipid profiles (cholesterol levels).

Research on cold-water specific therapy also clearly documents its benefit for decreasing pain, increasing heart rate variability, and for its effects on the normalization of sympathetic nerve activity, which has been shown to balance the stress responses (Higgins, Greene, & Baker, 2017).

NATUROPATHIC WISDOM

Water Therapy and My Physical Rehabilitation

Once I began my healing journey, I quickly learned that to regain my health, I needed to find an effective way to move. But the more I engaged with a physical therapist or tried to exercise on my own, the more pain I felt. For me, it seemed that everything I tried contracted and tightened the muscles in my neck and upper spinal column, which exacerbated my pain and drastically increased my nerve related symptoms. Finally, with the help of a sympathetic physical therapist, I decided to try swimming.

Covered in hives and barely able to walk from the dressing room to the pool without tipping over and falling in, when I first entered the water, I nearly drowned! Even with ten years of on-and-off physical therapy, both I and my therapist were truly shocked to learn how poor even my most basic sensory and vestibular (balance) functions were. In the pool, I could not even orient up from down if water got into my eyes. So, in that first attempt to swim (I had been a lifeguard and swam often when young so felt falsely comfortable swimming), I made it only halfway across a single lap of the pool until my physical therapist had to swim out and rescue me.

Today I can swim an average of sixty laps (in about sixty minutes), three times per week. Building to this level obviously took both time and effort. But as I rebuilt and rewired my body through swimming, I got my life back.

Chapter 14

I can now walk with little noticeable impairment, even though I still can't feel my right leg, I have plenty of physical stamina to do most anything that I want to do, I rarely feel like I can't catch my breath, and swimming keeps the nerve pain from my spinal cord injury in check. Because I swim using five different strokes, I also get a full-body workout that has, over time, coordinated and strengthened my muscle movements. Furthermore, I also get a 'swimmers high' that releases numerous beneficial endorphins which calm my anxiety and wash away my stress. In fact, when I am in the pool, I am more clear-headed than I ever am on land. For me, both the movement obtained within swimming and the therapeutic aspects of regularly being in water saved me.

Recommendations for Water-Based Therapies for Kids

In my experience, simply floating in warm water can be relaxing beyond description. For kids with high stress responses and anxiety, or for those reporting sensory overload, I often recommend time at a pool, in off hours, to simply float around and play in the water. This has proven especially beneficial for the kids in my practice who are having trouble sleeping. To specifically address sleep, I usually suggest visiting the pool after dinner has settled and before bed.

NATUROPATHIC WISDOM

For the kids I see, I also frequently suggest warm-water, evening baths, often with a drop or two of essential oil (I usually stick with lavender) and a single cup of Epsom salts. I have also found that warm-water baths in a dimly lit room are particularly beneficial when stabilizing a client who is in crisis or feeling extremely elevated levels of stress. For children who feel mildly suicidal or who are on the verge of a severe mental health crisis, I recommend two or three baths, every 24 hours, combined with plenty of sleep, lots of water to drink, and nutritious foods available to eat whenever the child feels hungry, around the clock. Within this protocol, I have kept a respectable number of my clients out of psychiatric hospitals (this method must also be accompanied by extremely careful and round-the-clock parental monitoring when suicidal ideation is a symptom).

According to Hussain and Cohen (2018) both steam-rooms and saunas also help the body to release impurities. So, for the kids I see who are suffering from numerous food sensitivities or allergies, and for those who are coming off a long run of prescription medication use, I often suggest 'sweating it out,' to the degree that is safe and approved for children and teens. I will add here that at most autism conferences, at least one infrared sauna salesperson is at the conference to detail the positive effects of the sauna for children with autism. Without going into specific details on why this method can be effective, the body of research suggests that one can mitigate some of the more deleterious effects seen in severe autism spectrum disorders by treating chemical sensitivities through detoxification and excretion within steam rooms and saunas (Pall, 2009).

When children sustain minor injuries, most people already know that water compresses (towels soaked in hot or cold water), can be used to alleviate pain and treat minor bruises and sprains. I also know personally that warm-water compresses placed directly on the chest can ease minor colds and speed up the release of mucous in the lungs; my grandmother taught me this.

In my experience, rigorous swimming and pool exercises are also good for kids. In fact, I have found that for a fair number of the kids I see, especially those who have refused to participate in other exercises or team sports, being on a swimming team or swimming solo for exercise is something they might consider.

Last, balneotherapy (soaking in mineral waters or hot springs) and thalassotherapy (spending time swimming in and absorbing the minerals of the ocean) are also recommended whenever these opportunities are possible. While there may yet be much left to learn about the healing benefits of at least certain waters, according to Moss (2010), it seems that time spent in water, especially time soaking or exercising in mineral springs and in the waters of the ocean is time well spent both for the healing of our minds and our bodies.

CHAPTER 15

Touch, Massage, and Acupressure for Kids

Chapter 15

"**S**ocial touch is a powerful force in human development, shaping social reward, attachment, cognitive, communication, and emotional regulation from infancy and throughout life" (Carissa, Cascio, Moore, & McGlone, 2019, p. 5). It is also known that severe developmental delay can occur when children do not receive normal touch and sensory stimulation from their caregivers (Ardiel & Rankin, 2010).

While most forms of touch are natural, and even spontaneous, when touch is planned, structured, and administered with the specific intent of healing, then that touch is said to have become therapeutic (Metzger, 2022, November). Touch therapy takes a variety of forms, but two of the most common of these are massage therapy and acupressure. Within these methods, using only one's hands, most parents can learn to provide basic therapeutic touch for their children.

Safe Touch and Touch Permission

Unfortunately, in our modern world, no responsible conversation about touch or touch therapy should move forward without a discussion first about the importance of teaching and enforcing safe touch. In the United States, approximately 28 percent of all children experience sexual assault before their sixteenth birthday, with the most common age for these assaults occurring between the ages of seven and thirteen (Finkelhor, 2010).

In my practice, to address these concerns, I provide information about a variety of 'safe touch' training programs. Having used several of these through the years, one program that I feel worthy of mention is the *Safe Touches Sexual Abuse Prevention Program for Children*. According to the Safe Touches website (2022), the program is an evidence-based training program that provides both school- and home-based support. Within a *My Body Belongs to Me* activity booklet, families and primary care givers complete various activities with their children to reinforce safe touch across all settings of a child's life. Through these shared activities, parents and caregivers not only reinforce lessons taught, but also open communication channels with their children so that children feel safe and comfortable discussing these topics in the years ahead (New York Society for the Prevention of Cruelty to Children, 2022).

In addition to safe touch training for younger children, I also encourage all parents to tell their children that **no adult outside of our family should be touching you anywhere on your body when there are no other children or adults present.** This statement alone, while not perfect, seems to provide a good 'rule-of-thumb' for most young families. For teachers and mental health therapists, I also recommend keeping doors open when meeting alone with children and only offering touch in the form of the 'side hug' or the 'pat on the back' between teachers and students. Unfortunately, to me this also means that teachers and mental health therapists who are not specifically licensed to administer massage therapy or acupressure should put their hands on a child. The administration of any massage or acupressure techniques with the children they serve, unless they are specifically given permission by both the child and the child's parents, and the specifics of these are formally detailed (in writing) within a student's individualized learning plan, should be avoided.

For pre-teens and teens, I have found that open and honest discussions about sexuality and intimacy are the most important deterrents to early sexual activity and sexual abuse prevention. But as this relates to the topic of this chapter, unfortunately, as we have also seen in the world of professional gymnastics, for example, coaches and others have specifically abused children under the guise of 'giving a sports massage.' So, I believe that specific discussions about massage need to occur with all youth who work with coaches or trainers who might have specific reasons to put their hands on a child or teen.

Simply put, with so many real threats out there, both kids and the adults who serve and teach them must be especially careful and diligent about: 1) the use of touch; and 2) the interpretation of how touch is delivered and perceived by the child. This is true whether touch is inadvertently given or delivered therapeutically. That said, there are still good ways for a teacher or therapist to provide information and model safe-touch and therapeutic techniques for self-application, and for use by parents so that children can explore the benefits of using massage therapy and acupressure on themselves and within their family.

The Use of Acupressure and Massage in a School Setting

Within the first few days of my brain injury, and still occasionally to this day, when my head trauma symptoms were at their worst, I instinctively pressed my thumbs deep into the palms of my hand. Most times when this happened. I was not even aware that I was doing this until someone pointed it out to me. For one of my early head injury doctors, this alone was the telltale sign that I had indeed suffered a traumatic brain injury; this behavior is common for those who have sustained brain trauma. Not long after I started doing this for myself, I also instinctively learned to calm my stomach and steady my balance by putting pressure on the front side of my wrists, about two inches above the joint, between the tendons. I also benefited from weekly massage therapy appointments to help me heal from my injuries and manage my pain.

Chapter 15

In looking back, I find it interesting that with no formal training at all, in either massage therapy or acupressure, I began to use two common pressure points to calm and steady myself. As I used these for myself, I also apparently began to use these same pressure points to calm the students in my school.

In fact, I did this so often that whenever certain children saw me, they would hold out their hands, as they sought out my administration of pressure at these points. For my students, I also began applying gentle pressure on the top of the head, although this was never something I practiced on myself; somewhere along the line, I found that this too calmed many kids.

In my school, we also had a 'peace place' where kids could use a large, three-nodule, massage therapy style vibrator on themselves and/or take a foot bath in one of several massaging foot bath stations. These were used along with heated weight bags, a variety of soft-bristle brushes, stretchy body socks that kids could crawl inside, and even a large, ground-level trampoline and ball pit.

In looking back, I now believe that many of the methods that we were calling 'sensory integration practices' doubled for self-administered massage therapy and acupressure work; there are a lot of crossovers between these fields. Irrespective of what we called these, I believe that children can use a variety of self-administered accommodations to learn how to self-regulate, calm down, relax sore muscles, improve

NATUROPATHIC WISDOM

focus, and step forward into a lifelong, personal self-care journey. Unfortunately, in far too many schools, not only are children not allowed these basic self-help accommodations, but even their basic needs to use the bathroom or eat when they are hungry are ignored 'until the bell rings.' We cannot teach children how to self-regulate and manage their own anxieties and difficulties with attention until we can openly let them explore the techniques that work to help them in these areas. For this reason, I believe that teaching children to self-deliver massage and acupressure is an easy first step at teaching self-awareness and self-control.

Historical Perspectives and Methodologies in Massage and Acupressure

The shared histories of massage therapy and acupressure date back thousands of years, with evidence suggesting that like other practices under the naturopathic umbrella, the practice of massage was present in Ancient Egypt, and early Chinese civilizations first began using acupressure around 2000 B.C. As both methods expanded, Hindu, Japanese, and Roman societies recognized and employed the practices, with modifications occurring across each society. Despite societal adaptations of the techniques, from ancient times until present day, both practices have retained their essential early characteristics and initial definitions. For massage, the practice is defined as 'the manipulation of the soft tissues of the body to enhance health and well-being.' Acupressure is defined as 'the treatment of symptoms by applying pressure with the fingers to specific pressure points on the body based on the Chinese system of energy flow across the body's meridians.' In Western culture, acupressure was first introduced in the 1600s, while massage therapy practices didn't make a formal appearance until the early 1800s.

According to Benjamin and Tappan (2005) and as detailed in their book *The Handbook of Healing and Massage Techniques*, massage therapy employs the use of effleurage (circular stroking movements), petrissage (kneading movements), friction (rubbing strokes), vibration (shaking movements to loosen up the body), and tapotement (tapping). Within these popular variations in how the massage therapy is delivered today, according to the American Massage Therapy Association (2022), popular adaptations of these methods include: Swedish Massage (the most widely recognized and commonly used type of massage); Deep Tissue Massage (which uses more pressure than the Swedish massage); Sports Therapy Massage (used in an athletic context to prevent injuries, improve recovery time, and enhance performance); Chair Massage (massage of the upper body, while fully clothed and seated in a special portable chair); and Trigger Point Massage (which employs a combination of light strokes and deep pressure to focus on areas of tight muscle fibers). Many massage therapists also draw from research in reflexology, the scientific study of lymphatic drainage, India's Ayurvedic medical approach, traditional Chinese Medicine, and the Japanese method of massage (Shiatsu). In addition, aromatherapy is also frequently used, and botanicals are also added to massage therapy oils in modern-day massage therapy.

In acupressure the therapist employs the use of 'finger pressure' to apply firm deep pressure (to the point of mild discomfort for the patient) to stimulate various 'pressure points' on the ears, hands, and feet. Drawing from the Chinese system of acupuncture, which has been shown to activate 'meridians or zones of energy flow for healing,' the acupressure therapist works to stimulate energy by activating these same points through pressure alone (without the use of needles). When stimulating pressure points on the ears, the acupressure therapist may use a fingernail, a pencil eraser, or even a matchstick to specifically target a specific pressure point. For pressure points in the hands and feet, the acupressure therapist usually uses a thumb to apply the pressure needed for activation of the targeted pressure point. Using this approach, practitioners have treated a wide variety of medical conditions simply by applying pressure to the associated pressure points relating to that body part, organ, or body system (Kenyan, 1988).

Chapter 15

The Research Supporting These Techniques

For massage therapy, both children and adults can benefit, with research findings supporting reduced anxiety, reduced aggressive behavior, pain reduction, improved sleep, improved attention and focus, better digestion and elimination, and increased motor functioning (Moyer, Rounds, & Hannum, 2004). In child-specific studies, where parents employed the techniques with their children, increased parent-child bonding is also a documented benefit (Gurol & Polat, 2012).

For acupressure, according to those who have clinically examined both acupuncture (a technique where these same pressure points are stimulated with a small, sterile needle) and acupressure, both methods appear to have the ability to stimulate the body's hormonal, circulatory, and lymphatic systems to relieve stress and anxiety, improve sleep, relax muscles and joints, regulate digestive issues, minimize headaches and migraines, and help with back pains and menstrual cramps. But in formal clinical studies, while acupuncture has been shown to significantly affect the above conditions, these effects appear "less well pronounced" in acupressure (Au, Tsang, Ling, Leung, and Cheung, 2015). However, in one randomized clinical trial that specifically examined acupressure alone within the post-operative surgical environment, both nausea and perceptions of pain were significantly reduced using only an acupressure technique (Unulu, M. & Nurten, K., 2017).

Massage Therapy for Kids

According to most massage therapy groups, massage can be used for children at a variety of different ages. Massage Therapists add that for young children, massage can even be used to teach anatomy. So, within the game of 'where's your foot?' young children can be gently introduced to massage and can even learn how to 'return massage' to parents within the use of games, which include rhythm, tapping activities, and songs. For school-aged children, massage can be delivered by parents to help children relax and calm down for work or sleep. Within the techniques used at this age, massage therapists suggest alternating pressure on the orbital bones of the eyes, using joint compressions such as the ones employed by occupational therapists, and beginning to teach children how to massage themselves on their hands, face, and feet. For touch-sensitive preteens and teens, practitioners suggest sticking to massage on the hands and feet, with offers to massage specific muscles in the neck, shoulders, and back that may feel sore or tight. Therapists treating teens also propose rolling on foam rollers for self-massage. While children and adults of all ages can benefit from professional massage therapy sessions, the pre-teen and teenage group are more likely to benefit from scheduled, thirty-minute massage therapy sessions with professional massage therapists.

Acupressure for Children and Teens

For acupressure, because the field of meridians and pressure points that are possible is so vast, I have chosen to include specific details for only seven of the primary pressure points that have demonstrated the most evidence for their effectiveness with children, either through clinical studies or from the reports of those who are in professional practice. Using points specifically found in the hands and feet, I feel parents can safely explore the following pressure points with their children. At each of the pressure points proposed below, apply small deep circles of pressure (should be firm and even a bit uncomfortable but not truly painful) for approximately fifteen to thirty seconds, then release. All pressure points are listed by their translated Chinese name (when that is available) and/or by their meridian and location number as assigned on a Chinese acupressure meridians chart. The seven points that I feel are worth exploring follow:

1. Called the Yin tang point, which is located on the forehead at about an inch above the eyebrows on the center of the face, this point can be stimulated to calm

the mind and may also help with focus and attention. I have used both tapping and pressure at this point.

2. The PC6 point, which is located on the wrist, three fingers below the inside center, appears to relieve hiccups, and acid reflux. This point is also said to calm the mind. In my experience, this point also calms a child who is hyperactive.

3. LI4, which is located along the top of the head has shown benefits for teething, neck pain, and toothache. This same LI4 meridian can also be found between the thumb and pointer finger on the hand. I apply pressure across this point, two or three times in succession (about two seconds of pressure then release and repeat), and this seems to help children calm and focus.

4. SP6, which is in the center of the ankle, three fingers from the inner ankle bone, can be used to help with sleep disturbances, anxiety, gas, and for constipation. I have students apply pressure here for themselves whenever they have tummy troubles.

5. LI11, located on the outside of the arm at the crease of the elbow, can reduce a low-grade fever, although I have not had personal experience with this particular pressure point.

6. Called the Bigger Rushing at Lv3, this point can be found between the foot bones of the first and second toe and helps with leg cramps and lower body

growing pains. I have found this point good for any pain in the lower body.

7. Pericardium 6, which is located between the two tendons on the inside of the wrist, approximately an inch above the joint, may calm the mind while also easing an upset stomach. As a side note, interestingly, pressure on this point has also been developed for use in motion-sickness therapies with the use of the 'sea band,' which replaces thumb pressure with a plastic button that can be pressed for nausea. I have used sea bands to additionally help kids with anxiety.

CHAPTER 16

Nutrition and Healthy Eating

Chapter 16

Clearly, no book covering even the most basic aspects of naturopathy would be complete without a discussion on the benefits of a healthy and nutritious diet. I am also a mom of two grown-up picky eaters, and as such, I know that especially as it relates to nutrition with children and teens, kids do not always eat the food in front of them. So, while I do intend to share suggestions on what constitutes good nutrition, I am going to first talk about some of the real problems that underly the subject of why kids do not eat healthy food.

In two examples for my own children, my daughter who was always quite sensitive to gluten lived on bagels and cream cheese for the better part of her senior year in high school, and my son, who is now twenty-eight years old, told me just a few weeks ago that he was finally feeling better because he came to the realization that he could not "live on Taco Bell and bourbon." You can't make this stuff up! So, before I dive into any discussion about how you as a parent could work harder to prepare even more nutritious food for your family, I will first address the real-world challenge of getting kids to eat. Let's start by talking about some of the research-based reasons that kids do not eat.

NATUROPATHIC WISDOM

Children Are Not Little Adults
When It Comes to Food

First, children are not little adults. According to Mennella and Bobowski (2015), children's taste buds are biologically quite different from those of adults, and they have more of them. These differences cause them to seek sweets, which helps babies desire their mothers' milk, and avoid bitter or overly sour foods, which prevents babies and young children from eating things that are toxic. This means that for children, many foods do taste different. Remember when you were a kid? Weren't there foods that you hated then but eat regularly now? The actual taste of many foods dramatically changes in flavor as we age and as our taste buds mature. These include obvious foods within the cruciferous food category, such as cabbage, broccoli, spinach, and brussels sprouts, as well as the sour or bitter flavors of lemons and grapefruit. Tomatoes also change in taste quite dramatically from childhood to adulthood. But because of their increased number of taste buds, children may also be sensitive to other foods too, and these can include foods that are salty, spicy, or fermented in their flavor. In short, our sense of taste matures to be less sensitive throughout our lifetimes.

Children also have far less maturity in knowing their taste and food preferences So, taste, smell, texture, and even the sounds made, or the pressure required to chew up food causes children to rely much more heavily on visual appearance when approaching unfamiliar foods (Chung & Fong, 2018). This means that when eating, the way that foods look (their visual familiarity) also becomes critical in developing kids' food choices. Children have a much harder time eating foods that look, smell, or taste unusual.

Taste Preference is Acquired Over Time

Next, our taste preferences have been shown to develop in the first few years of our lives, and for most kids today, these early taste preferences have been developed within processed baby foods and from food 'treats.' When my kids were little, they only tolerated three or four distinct types of baby food each, and, tired of throwing others out, I bought the ones they liked and stuck to what worked. I suspect others did and still do the same.

But within the entire Gerber line of baby food products (which was then and still is a leading baby food line), the full range of food flavors possible, according to the Gerber food website (2022, November) includes: apple, avocado, banana, beef, blueberry, carrot, cereal, and chicken. There were even fewer options in years past. As you can see, there is not much here in the way of leafy green things. The reason for this is obvious: these foods are easy to digest, well tolerated, and they all taste quite bland. But it is also helpful to know that within most manufactured baby food lines, these early foods also contain added sugar, salt, and fat. In this way, babies acquire specific and limited taste preferences before they are even weaned from baby food (Riley, 2019).

I am not suggesting that we try to give babies and toddlers mashed-up spinach. I suspect we know how that would go. But I am providing this information to remind us how most children's tastes develop. So as parents, we often need to gently expand on our children's early taste preferences soon after weaning them from baby food if we expect them to eat differently in their teens.

Sugar and Fast-Delivery Carbohydrates Are Addictive

Next, it is helpful to note that fast-delivery carbohydrates, such as white bread, pasta, and the like (which break down quickly as simple sugars in the body) and the actual consumption of sugars are known to be physically and neurochemically addictive. According to Avena, Rada, and Hoebel (2008), when we consume sugar or carbohydrates that quickly turn into sugar, or consume actual sugar, our bodies release trace amounts of opioids and dopamine with addictive potential. These opioids are compounded further when poorly digested gluten and casein (milk proteins) are combined.

Chapter 16

Especially when eating foods high in sugar, such as candy and soda pop, these can cause the classical behaviors of binging, withdrawal, cravings, and the buildup of increased tolerance, which mirrors the neurochemical changes in the brain that occur with addictive drug use (Wiss, Avena, & Rada. 2018). But here is a crucial point—intermittent withholding of simple carbohydrates and sugars, then binging on them later is far worse for creating these addictive patterns than simply having access to smaller amounts of these sugars. For some of the kids I see, especially for those who have had all sugars and fast-delivery carbohydrates withheld, but with access to these in other settings (because kids can usually still access sugar when their parents are not around), sugar cravings can become so intense that parents are forced to hide actual sugar so that children don't sit and eat it with a spoon. I have even observed a child who stole handfuls of sugar packets from the school lunchroom to feed these cravings.

This suggests that when we intermittently withhold sugar and fast-delivery sugar/carbohydrates, then we give in to these, or children and teens access these outsides of the home, which we often cannot control, children can and do become 'addicted' to the neurochemical responses.. This can result in seeking, hoarding, and binging behaviors (Avena, Bartley, & Hoebel, 2012). So rather than attempting to withhold all sugars and fast-delivery carbohydrates in the home, because they are so readily available everywhere else, we must instead teach our children how to manage their sugar and carbohydrate consumption, in moderation, and for their own wellness.

While babies are biologically primed when young to crave anything that is even slightly sweet for survival, in the past, once we were old enough to start eating adult foods, there was little true sugar available in nature. So, sweets and carbohydrates came primarily from fruits and whole grains. But as worldwide food industries grew, sweetened fruits and grains, stripped of their natural fibers (which speeds up the conversion from carbohydrate to sugar), and sugar-enhanced foods were mass-produced, which led to an increased demand for sweets in people of all ages and across the globe. As these demands grew, food production entities responded by increasing the amount of added sugar in foods, and many societies began eating as much sugar as they could get, which still was not much until only one hundred years ago. But today, and with the introduction of high fructose corn syrup and other highly condensed sugars (which are especially bad sugars because they fool the tongue by not tasting overly sweet) more available and less expensive to produce, added sugars (in staggering amounts) are present in a variety of everyday foods. Added sugars are especially common, because they are less expensive than other more nutritious ingredients in the things we drink. So now, milk, natural fruit juice, and even water is replaced by sweetened juice and soft drinks in many homes. According

Chapter 16

to White (2018) within these trends, sugar consumption has risen 1000% in only the past one hundred years (that is not a type error). While we all could work together to reduce our sugar consumption habits, it is important to remember that our kids crave these even more than we do as adults, and these are available everywhere. Rather than trying to eliminate sugar entirely from our children's diet, we may need to draw from what we know about sugar's addictive properties to help our children learn the skill of proper sugar consumption.

Food Access, Food Sensitivities, and Food Control

As another reason that many children do not eat healthy food, there is also the real problem that nutritious food has become increasingly more expensive to purchase, prepare, and deliver when compared to highly processed, overly refined, and sugar, fat, and salt-rich food. In fact, in America, 33.8 million Americans (10.4 percent) live in households that struggle with access to an affordable, nutritious diet, according to the Food Research and Action Center (2022). While food assistance programs help, these are often forced to focus on delivering 'shelf-stable bulk foods,' which tend to be those foods that are more processed and less dense in nutrition.

181

NATUROPATHIC WISDOM

In my work with clinical allergists, I have learned that we also tend to crave the very foods we are allergic or chemically sensitive to. In fact, one pediatric allergist that I know can correctly guess a child's food allergies by simply listing the top ten foods that the child prefers to eat. According to Cutler (2010), a child's allergies and food sensitivities are usually present on a child's top ten favorite foods list. Why is this true? Apparently when a child eats food that they are mildly allergic or sensitive to, the resultant histamine response that occurs in the body triggers the release of endorphins that, while necessary to protect the body from harm, also feel good. These endorphins keep kids coming back to the foods to which they are mildly allergic.

For the last of the major reasons why I believe kids do not eat, I broach a much more difficult topic by stating that certain children have the budding characteristics of eating disorders, even when they are quite young. In my practice, I have seen kids who choose not to eat as a means of control, to try to lose weight, to feel the adrenal effects of low blood sugar, and so they can eat, purge, and eat again. I also know that severe challenges with eating are present for some clients with developmental disabilities, such as autism, because for these kids, sensory sensitivities combine with poor digestive health to compound the issues listed above.

Chapter 16

To give you an idea about what these might look like, I can count at least four different and unrelated children in my practice who eat only Cheerios (and have done so for several years).

Parents Want to Feed Their Children Healthy Food

With so many reasons for kids to not eat healthy, it really should not surprise us that some kids do not eat the healthy well-balanced meals that their parents try to prepare for them. Let me reinforce that point: I rarely see parents who do not know how to or do not have the desire to feed their children properly. In fact, just for fun, I did a quick Google search with the "all intext:" feature for keywords "children," "nutrition," and "books" (within this feature all three terms must be included in the search), and as of November 2022, there have been over eight million books published on the topic of children's nutrition! This tells me that parents are well-read, they want to feed their children healthy food, and there is no shortage of literature on how to prepare a healthy and nutritious diet for children. With that in mind, I will not attempt to write another children's nutrition chapter here. But I will share my own experiences, and I will draw lines of similarity between the most well-accepted dietary trends in use today.

NATUROPATHIC WISDOM

The USDA Food Pyramid

When we were kids, every school classroom contained a picture of the USDA food pyramid. For those who have never seen this, I will describe it as it was burned into my memory. The pyramid had four levels. Grains were at the bottom for six to eleven servings per day (no, I am not kidding). Fruits and vegetables shared the next level with a recommended four to six servings of vegetables and two to three servings of fruit recommended each day. The next level included a combination of all dairy products, protein, and seed and nut sources, with two to three servings of dairy and meat recommended daily (the nuts and seeds were just in the picture). At the very top of the pyramid was a small triangle that stated fats, oils, and sweets 'should be used sparingly.' Within these guidelines, most parents tried to comply, and this meant that as children, we ate as many grains as we could eat.

Recall that this was the era in which most children in America began their day with a bowl of sweetened cereal, a glass of sweetened fruit juice, and a piece of white-bread toast with sweetened jelly. Lunch was often another two slices of bread with some kind of meat and cheese or peanut butter and another serving of sweetened jelly, as most kids ate a sandwich and a piece of fruit for lunch. Dinner for most was a meat and potatoes affair, with another serving of bread or rolls accompanying the main dish, a small

Chapter 16

salad or side of vegetables, and usually a dessert. Within these eating trends, diabetes, obesity, and heart disease exploded. But cereal companies still aggressively competed for consumer dollars and spent considerable effort in those days to get us hooked on our favorite cereal. Along with increasingly sweetened grains that were reinforced with toys, games, riddles, they baited us with kid-friendly short stories about various animals, people, or science which covered the cereal box. One year, my brother and I were even elated to learn that we had won a treasure chest containing 100 different board games. We waited eagerly for this chest to arrive. When it came, the entire prize was folded into an 8-inch by 10-inch envelope and building the 'treasure chest' was one of the games that we could make ourselves with various tiny pieces of pre-cut cardboard and plastic. I remember knowing then that the cereal companies were conning us. Luckily, my brother and I were shielded from some of the most severe problems with eating overly sweetened cereal first thing in the morning, as our parents usually tried to make us eat fruit cocktail and scrambled eggs with a slice of homemade bread; and we always drank a glass of whole milk. But instead of simply eating cereal for breakfast, we frequently snuck in a bowl of cereal after school or on the weekend when they were not looking.

That food pyramid today has been modified to what is now called the FDA Plate, which shows that the construction of a healthy plate at any meal should include two larger portions of grains and vegetables, two slightly smaller portions of protein and fruit, and a small round circle on the side of the plate (about the size of a glass) to suggest the recommended consumption of dairy at each meal. So even today, the food guidelines provided by the FDA are not clear about how much to eat or what exactly we should be eating. This has left a vacancy filled by various fad diets, which has led to even more confusion.

Healthy Eating Can Be Confusing

So, what exactly is the healthiest diet? Over the past fifty years, I have seen dozens of changes in dietary recommendations, some of these even complicating things so much that as a young mother I remember feeling like I could not feed my kids anything without making some mistake in healthy eating. Throughout my life, within various diets, I have been told that sugar and carbohydrates were bad, meat was bad, most nuts were bad, beans were bad, many fruits were bad, dairy was bad, eggs were bad, fat was bad, and salt was bad. In my mind, this left me with only a handful of good fruits and unsalted vegetables, of which potatoes, corn, carrots, and peas were bad because they contained too many carbohydrates. As a young mom who wanted to do everything right, this list of bad foods left me with a lengthy list of questions and short list of healthy food.

Chapter 16

By the time I tried to eliminate everything that some dietician or other had reported as bad, and with almost nothing left to actually eat, there was one point where I had the temptation to just give up and feed my kids whatever they wanted, as it was certainly easier than keeping track of all the 'bad food rules.' Especially in the 1990s, contradictory food information was enough to drive a person insane, because obviously, not everything we eat can be bad.

It was then that I began to seriously do food research on my own, and with the help of a friend who was a nutritionist, I learned that most natural, whole foods, when eaten in moderation, can and should be included in a healthy diet. This means that a wide variety of fruits, vegetables, nuts, seeds, legumes, whole grains, low-fat meats, low-fat dairy products, eggs, and good added fat sources such as olive oil can all be combined to create a healthy, well-rounded diet.

Healthy Eating Habits that We Can All Agree On

Today, and with still little clarity from the FDA, there are still dozens of common dietary trends that are in use. According to the *US News and World Report* (2022), the most common diets across the eating spectrum include various Vegetarian and Vegan diets, the Mediterranean, DASH, and Flexitarian diets, the Paleo diet, and various low-carbohydrate diets such as the Ketogenic and Atkins diets. While these vary quite considerably in how foods are combined, or even regarding which foods should be included or avoided, within all of these, surprisingly, there are some universal threads that lay solid groundwork for good, common-sense eating habits. So rather than disputing which diet is healthiest or argue with someone who is entirely vegan vs. a family who has chosen to eat a lot of meat and protein at the exclusion of certain grains and fruits, I'll draw a line through what I see as the common-sense middle ground within the most utilized dietary trends in use today. I believe that in so doing, I can safely share a basic framework for healthy eating habits.

First, it appears that a diet rich in plant-based foods that includes a wide variety of different vegetables and fruits (especially those with lower sugar/carbohydrate content) should make up the largest portion of the diet (Medawar, Huhn, Villringer, & Veronica Witte, 2019). Certainly (and obviously when kids eat them), leafy green and cruciferous vegetables such as spinach, broccoli, kale, cauliflower, and cabbage are all great choices, and these should be consumed heavily across all diets. Ideally, at least a handful of fruits and vegetables should be from an organic source, if possible, as some of these contain high amounts of pesticides. According to the 'Dirty Dozen Food Lists' (Winter & Katz, 2011), especially for young children, strawberries, apples, celery, peaches, nectarines, bell peppers, grapes, and cherries appear to bear the most residue.

Chapter 16

Next (and depending some on the dietary preference), various nuts, seeds, and legumes, especially those with lower carbohydrate counts and healthier fat content, are recommended across all diets (Afshin, Micha, Khatibzadeh, & Mozaffarian, 2014). Across current dietary trends, it is well-accepted that almonds are the healthiest nut. From there, other tree nuts (cashews, walnuts, pecans, etc.) are deemed healthier than bush nuts (peanuts). Various healthy seeds can also be drawn from a variety of sources, and pumpkin, chia, and sunflower seeds are especially healthy (de Souza, Schincaglia, Pimentel, & Mota, 2017).

In diets where meat is consumed, meat that is lower in fat, fresh, or frozen fresh, and less commercially processed is always recommended as the best choice. Across meat-eating diets, there are also recommendations to eat meat that is less polluted with growth hormones and chemical preservatives, when these are available. Dieticians across all trends also agree that certain fish, such as wild-caught salmon, may be especially healthy. In short, across the various meat-eating diets, selected meat should be in its cleanest and leanest state and eaten in moderation (Richi, Baumer, Conrad, Darioli, Schmid, & Keller, 2015).

Next, across all common diets in use today, at least some grains are consumed, and the selection of these is recommended to be those that are the least refined and the most complex in their fiber and protein content (McRae, 2017). In diets where grains feature more heavily, certain natural, organically grown grains are suggested, when possible, to avoid the potential disruptive digestive factors associated with consuming larger quantities of pesticides and herbicides (Myers, et al., 2016). For those who are sensitive to or cannot tolerate wheat, as is the case in the autoimmune-based disorder of Celiac Disease, a variety of plant- and nut-based flours and non-wheat grains now can take the place of the complex and otherwise nutritious wheat grain (Saturni, Ferretti, & Bacchetti, 2010). However, when eating grains, even in their complex and natural form, it is important to know that these ultimately convert to carbohydrates (sugars) in the body. So, a good rule for grains is this: the slower the grain is to digest, the better it is for the body, assuming the body can effectively digest the grain and the grain does not just sit and ferment in the digestive system. All dieticians also agree that highly processed and overly refined grains that have been stripped of their fiber are not good for the body.

Dairy products and eggs are also included, in moderation, in most healthy eating plans (except for the purely vegan diet). Here the mix of carbohydrates and fats that are present within different milk-based products appears to be the primary consideration between the various diets, with some disagreement about using whole dairy or fat-free dairy across the research (Bakke, Shehan, & Hayes, 2016). There are mixed findings within the research to suggest that the added nutrition within whole egg and whole dairy products may or may not be fully offset by the problems introduced with the increased fats that these whole products contain. All diets that do consume dairy recognize a rising trend to substitute goat milk and nut-based milk and cheese products, at least at times, as cow-based dairy substitutes, as these are often easier to digest and lower in saturated fats. Eggs, which are discussed within a category of their own in various diets, are also consumed in many diets, as these are heavily packed with nutrition. But here too, there is still no consensus about whether the fat in an egg yolk is nutrition-ally well-balanced or whether the egg should be modified by eating the white of the egg only. Across all dairy and egg discussions, focus on the cholesterol levels versus the nutritional components of the various forms of these foods when whole is the primary point of difference (Oakenfull & Sidhu, 1992).

Fat by itself is also an important aspect of discussion, with all agreeing that healthy, unsaturated Omega-3 fats (such as those found in olives, flax seeds, coconuts, and certain nuts), are needed in a healthy diet and these are far better for us than the more common Omega-6 saturated fats that are readily present in margarine, vegetable oil, and fried foods. When consuming fats, butter, animal, and vegetable fat can easily become problematic for those who eat larger quantities, and there is agreement that these too significantly raise cholesterol levels. So as a basic guide here, butter may still be better than margarine (I am recalling some

NATUROPATHIC WISDOM

TV commercials from my childhood with a smile here), but olive oil and certain nut oils are clearly better than either animal or dairy oils for the introduction of good fat into the diet (Liu et al., 2017).

Across all diets, added sugar and salt should be used sparingly, although synthetic, sugar-free substitutes are not necessarily less problematic than actual sugar (Tandel, 2011). Plant-based sweeteners such as stevia, along with raw, natural honey, appear to be the best sources of natural sweetness, along with unsweetened fruits (without added sugar). It should be noted here that honey should not be used raw for young children. On another note, because there are usually large quantities of added sugars, salt, and Omega-6 fat in many prepared foods, food condiments, fruit juices, sweetened yogurt, salad dressing, and canned prepared foods need to be monitored carefully for their sugar and/or salt content, as even when eating healthy, a glass of juice, a blob of ketchup, a side of yogurt, or a commercially prepared salad dressing could easily tip over an otherwise healthy meal (Ponzo et al., 2021).

In the past ten years, nutritionists have also pushed heavily for the re-introduction of naturally occurring digestive enzymes and probiotic-rich foods into the diet, such as the ones found in fermented foods. Soemarie, Milanda, and Barliana (2021) tell us that probiotic-rich foods such as kefir, tempeh, natto, kombucha, miso, kimchi, sauerkraut, and probiotic yogurt improve gut health by improving

Chapter 16

the immune system's ability to protect us from unhealthy 'pathogenic' bacteria. This makes sense if we think about it. All through our past, without food preservatives or good refrigeration methods, humans have eaten age-fermented foods. For the past fifty years or more, we have believed that the more sterile a food was, the better it was. But we are now beginning to understand that certain fermented foods strengthen the body in a variety of ways.

Children Learn Good Eating Habits from Their Parents

What, when, and how we eat is a highly personal choice. For children, eating is also one of the few things that they can truly control. But luckily, we also know that kids acquire most of their adult eating habits from their parents. This means that as the first and most important rule in teaching kids about healthy eating, we must model for them what healthy eating looks like. I still cook many of the same things that I ate when I lived at home with my own parents. So, the good news is this: even if your kids are not eating what you prepare now, they are still learning how to prepare healthy food for themselves when they become adults.

Within our own healthy eating, we should also try to expand on and introduce a variety of new food options for ourselves and for our kids while being patient when new food options are not immediately a hit. Poor nutrition occurs within all diets when we resort to eating only a small number of the same foods, day in and day out. To expand on what kids will eat, we should start by feeding kids what they will eat. Then slowly and gently we can introduce a variety of new foods. This does not mean that we should strive to prepare something new at every meal. Nor should we cook separate meals for different members of the family. The 'basic meal staple' can be a lifesaver. But we can increase interest and possibility when we approach new foods, as a family, with open-mindedness and curiosity. This can, in time, become a good approach to expanding on what our kids will eat, and it might mean that we need to even try out some of our kids' favorite foods too. Finally, because we all have about a dozen 'go-to' meals that we regularly prepare, I encourage parents to start a meal exchange program with other parents they know to borrow recipes and even sample another family's staple 'go-to' dinners. Families can also do 'potluck' dinners to expose children to new foods. Food sharing can be a fun way for parents to safely introduce new foods.

Kids are also more invested in eating healthy meals when they participate in their own meal preparation. In my experience, children benefit from learning how to cook basic meals for themselves and from helping with meal preparation for the family. I will add that I have heard about some priceless 'aha moments' when a child has worked hard to prepare a meal for the family and a younger sibling then complains about it or will not eat it.

Choice and Food Access

Within my line of work, I have arrived at the belief that kids should never be bribed, manipulated, or physically forced to eat things that they do not want to eat. I will add that the old saying "you may not leave the table until you have finished your food" usually does more harm than good. Forced or manipulated eating (either through reward or punishment) or by any show of threat or force often only sets children up for food-related control issues and eating disorders in adulthood. Also, when kids do not want to or don't feel they can eat the meal that has been prepared, they should not 'go to bed hungry' either; a reasonably healthy grab-and-go snack, meal replacement drink, or other ready-made meal alternative should be allowed. That said, encouraging children to taste and try new foods is not a terrible thing at all, and again, while I do not recommend that parents try to manipulate children into trying or tasting new foods, they can be gently encouraged.

Next, one straightforward way to help kids eat nutritious food is to simply buy, prepare, and keep nutritious food in the house. We all know that it is easier to grab small, ready-to-eat carrot sticks from a bag rather than clean, trim, and cut up a whole carrot. So having a wide variety of easy-to-eat nutritious snacks on hand and ready to eat makes it easier for kids to snack nutritiously. Also, for kids who refuse to eat the meal prepared, but later raid the pantry for highly processed food or sweets, these alternative food choices may need to be removed from the pantry entirely, for a time, until children can learn to better manage their eating choices.

Last, eating healthy should be an everyday occurrence. So, I do not recommend that parents buy sugary soft drinks, bulky sweets, or highly processed food snacks just for special events, parties, or when on vacation. When parents provide these foods as 'special treats' they are creating unhealthy associations between celebrating and eating poorly. I am not suggesting here that children go without a birthday cake or that they never have access to a bag of potato chips. I am instead saying that teaching children to associate eating healthy with celebrating is a better lifestyle choice. For this same reason, food should, in general, **not** be utilized to reward good behavior.

Among all these suggestions, common-sense middle ground is certainly necessary. I have observed that when children are never allowed to eat at least some of the same things that their peers are eating, they resort to sneaking and hoarding food. I have also known parents who have tried to indulge their child's food preference with the result of a teenager who only eats ramen noodles. In addition, not only is food choice a consideration, but when kids eat also needs to be discussed.

Special Considerations for Breakfast, Lunch, and Dinner

For the kids I work with, many have the most difficulty when eating either breakfast or lunch. To address challenges with eating breakfast I will say this—I am amazed by the things that creative parents have been able to get their kids to tolerate when blended into a breakfast smoothie. A good breakfast smoothie can start simply with just fresh or frozen fruit (berries over bananas are better due to sugar content), nut-based milk, and ice.

From here, parents can then experiment by adding tiny amounts of vegetables, healthy oils such as nut butters, protein powders, and even ground oatmeal (black berries and blueberries do a great job of hiding both the taste and color of these ingredients). When building breakfast smoothies, I usually recommend that parents start with something familiar that they know their child will drink. Then, very slowly, parents can add in additional healthy ingredients. Kids can also learn to experiment by creating their own smoothies. Last, for breakfast, while we should all try to avoid highly processed food when we can, there are several good breakfast bars that can be stored in the car or placed in a child's backpack for consumption on the way to school.

School lunch can also be an especially challenging time for some kids, even if kids pack their own lunch, because the time allotted in school to eat is short, and the sensory overload of being in a lunchroom often feels chaotic and disruptive for proper eating and digestion. So, for kids who tend to go all day without eating, I have found that a quieter lunch setting, such as an administrative office or even the student's classroom, may be needed (with a doctor's note this can be a legal accommodation) to improve eating during the day. Eating away from peers should not be used as a form of punishment for not eating, however. The quieter lunch space should only be used when kids specifically ask for it or agree to it. For kids who do not eat lunch at school, parents need to talk to their kids about why they are not eating and work with school personnel to figure out a solution. I have also found that for most kids who take stimulant medication, they simply cannot eat while medicated. For these kids, the calories missed during the day often need to be recovered in the evening.

Most kids are also ravenous at the end of a school day, but a heavy or filling snack at this time of day often disrupts hunger for dinner time. So after-school snacks should be light, and it is here that a faster, carbohydrate-rich energy boost can be a good thing. Far too often I see kids who eat a big 'snack-like meal' after school, then refuse more nutritious food at dinner.

Eating Healthy Is Challenging

For far too many reasons, a lot of today's kids are nutritionally deficient. Even within what should be considered 'healthy eating protocols,' the foods that kids eat in modern food production practices makes healthy eating difficult. We also know that even the soil in which food is grown is now more nutritionally depleted than it was fifty years ago. Simply put, the peach I ate as a child is not as nutritionally complete as the peach eaten just last week. For those of us who are older, we can even remember when many fruits and vegetables tasted different than they do today.

Within the lens of naturopathy, I could, therefore, tell you that you need to work harder to buy, prepare, and feed your children healthy and nutritious food, which may be true; I could add that you are failing your child by not feeding them a healthy, natural, whole-food diet. But facts are facts—even though commercially prepared food is more readily available than it has ever been before, feeding children with a nutritious and healthy diet is harder than ever before because there are so many unhealthy food alternatives. Therefore, as a second-best alternative for kids who will not eat well on their own, or for families who find it hard to feed their kids well, I recommend the use of a good, high-quality, children's multi-vitamin/mineral supplement, especially during periods of high stress. While this form of nutrition does not replace healthy eating, supplemental nutrition is certainly better than no nutrition at all.

When using supplements, as was recommended in the previous chapter on herbs and plants, I suggest supplements that are as close to their natural food source as is possible. In the vitamin and supplement world these are frequently referred to as 'whole food supplements,' and there are dozens of different options that can become overwhelming to the parent consumer. It is here then that a good nutritionist can guide you. While food supplementation sounds complicated, the good news is this: there are some excellent food supplement options available for children who will not eat what is needed for good health and are suffering from nutritional deficiencies. For children who over-eat, or binge eat, nutritional supplements have also been shown to decrease these patterns of eating. Researchers Anders and Schroeter (2017) explain this by stating that we tend to eat until our nutritional needs are met, despite hunger, but children are notoriously bad at knowing what they are lacking within the food they are eating, so they just keep eating. For this reason, over-eating also often suggests nutritional deficiency.

When kids will not eat or will not eat the foods that they need to sustain a healthy mind and body, I also recommend consultation with an integrative or biomedical doctor, a

Chapter 16

licensed naturopath, or a skilled nutritionist or dietician to build better food habits and rule out hidden food allergies. When eating or not eating becomes compulsive, mental health support is usually required. Last, for children with autism and other developmental disabilities specifically, there is a large body of research and support for healing the digestive system and building nutritional eating habits. These supports include food sensitivity testing, detoxification and cleansing diets, supplementing food with various food and mineral sources, and even cookbooks for the sensitive autistic eater.

When it comes to nutrition, I think the most important things to remember are these: kids need to eat healthy foods for the development of healthy minds and bodies. But there are lots of reasons why kids will not eat and attempting to force eating will not help. Kids are also remarkably resilient, and they can survive for quite a while on marginally nutritious food. Additionally, most children do eventually develop adequate food habits, and they draw these habits from the foods they ate as children. As they mature, they also learn what they like and start figuring out how certain foods make them feel; but this process can take a long time. Therefore, while modeling good eating practices is important, even if our kids choose to ignore these, resorting to supplements does not mean that we have failed; these may be necessary to get kids through difficult eating years. From my experience, I can also say that most kids do adopt better food habits as they mature. Parents should, therefore, not beat themselves up when their kids will not eat. Remember that even those of us who work in professional fields with children have kids that did not eat healthy at various points during their growing up years. Most kids who have normal physical and mental health development eventually learn that eating healthy feels good. Until then, we as parents must simply continue to do the best we can.

Last on this topic, and despite one's views on politics and/or food assistance programs, I fully recommend and support all programs that feed hungry children who are otherwise not able to secure healthy or nutritious food on their own. In my mind, even if we just look at this through the lens of the financial cost-to-benefit ratio to society, we are much wealthier as a society when all children can eat healthy and nutritious food. From where I stand, I see far too many kids who cannot eat the foods they need to be healthy. These same kids cannot think well, they cannot learn easily, and they cannot then contribute to the society in which they live. There is also nothing more heartbreaking than watching a child watch others eat in a school cafeteria, when their own lunch box is empty.

CHAPTER 17

Common-Sense Recommendations for Serious Mental Health Crises

Chapter 17

In my professional career, I have seen dozens of suicidal kids. I have also lost two teens that I knew personally to suicide. So, in this last chapter, even though it ends us on a heavy note, I would like to share a final personal story for the purpose of guiding parents through the process of figuring out what to do in a serious mental health crisis. Here, I will also remind everyone that there is a suitable time and place for the introduction and implementation of naturopathic interventions, and there is also a time to seek out trained, professional mental health and medical services that may include hospitalization. Before I begin, I will say that I debated long and hard on ending this work here. I considered leaving this out entirely and I considered following this with another chapter. But in the end, I finally came to this conclusion—a chapter on severe mental health and mental health crisis is desperately needed and this chapter also gives us some of the best examples for employing common sense when embarking on an alternative path of health and healing. Simply put, as naturopathy relates to addressing the mental health of children and teens, starting a path of naturopathic treatment, without other allopathic mental health or medical treatments, while in the thick of a serious mental health crisis is **never recommended**.

NATUROPATHIC WISDOM

My Depression and Lessons Shared

During the last three years of my illness, when I was most severely afflicted by poor health, and I had been taking five to ten prescription medications (on average) for over a decade, I suffered from true, clinical depression. In saying this I do not mean that I was sometimes sad, or that I cried too much. What I experienced (and had not properly understood before, even within all my clinical training) was that a very real and true biophysiological change had overtaken my normal thinking process. In this, I could not see a positive future for myself, I could not clearly think about myself in relationship to living a healthy, sustainable, or happy life, and over time, I had genuinely begun to think about ending things. In today's world we know that about 13 percent of all children and teens consider committing suicide before they turn eighteen (Becker, & Correll, 2020).

One day, with a large quantity of prescription pain killers assembled in one hand and my cellphone in the other, I made the decision to seek out much more intensive and professional help than I was getting from my various medical doctors. In a true crisis of my own, I made the hard decision to admit myself to the emergency room for mental health treatment. To do this, one must only go into a hospital and request a behavioral health assessment. For families who have a child in crisis, this can be one way to initiate immediate mental health intervention services. There is also a

Chapter 17

national mental health hotline that initiates immediate evaluation and treatment services when children or adults are experiencing a mental health crisis. Support for these can be accessed by simply dialing 988, and this route into treatment is recommended over calling the police, as the individuals involved have at least basic mental health training. Once a call to this number is made, a series of steps will be initiated that can include everything from talking a parent through the process until de-escalation has occurred to picking up a child and taking them to the hospital or nearby crisis center.

Once I self-admitted to the emergency room, a mental health worker conducted a crisis-risk threat assessment, and I was referred for inpatient psychiatric hospitalization. Because it took time for the doctors in the emergency room to find me a 'bed' I was kept in the ER until I could be transported to a psychiatric hospital. Here I will add that as soon as the threat assessment was complete, and my risk was determined to be concerning, I no longer retained the right to leave the hospital on my own or transport myself to a different facility; my admission to the hospital became mandatory for what is often referred to as the 'seventy-two-hour hold.'

I find it helpful to explain to the families I work with that this is a standard procedure whenever anyone is considered a serious risk to themselves or others. But this also means that there is legally nothing they, as parents, can do to get their child out of the emergency room or psychiatric facility in less than seventy-two hours, and transportation between facilities is usually overseen by hospital personnel or the police department. For some parents this alone can feel daunting, but here I remind parents that the alternative (taking the child home or transporting the child themselves) could potentially be much more dangerous. I also mention that medical and psychiatric staff at the hospital can release a child sooner if they feel the seventy-two-hour hold is not warranted, and in fact, a number of parents I know have been surprised by the call to come and pick up their child in as little as eight to twelve hours.

For me, I knew that I would give up many legal rights on admission. But in addition to addressing my suicidal thoughts, I also consciously made my decision to admit myself to the hospital specifically to gain access to more immediate psychiatric care. Several days before my trip to the ER, I had tried to get an appointment with a psychiatrist but was placed on a wait list that was approximately three months out. I knew I simply could not wait that long. Upon admission to the psychiatric facility, I did in fact meet with a licensed psychiatrist within seven hours of my admission to the hospital. While the timing of meeting with a psychiatrist can vary from state to state, for parents who are in severe crisis with their children, sometimes a hospital admission is the fastest (although not necessarily the best) route towards accessing immediate psychiatric care. Most advanced care mental-health placement centers, such as inpatient psychiatric hospitals, have a psychiatrist on staff, and psychiatric services are required for this level of hospital admission by most insurance carriers.

Once in the hospital, I knew I would also lose the right to control my own medical care. As an example, I was not allowed to take my birth control pills. This point does have exceptions, however, and I learned this when one of the weekend doctors referred me for electroconvulsive therapy (yes, shock therapy is still a thing for the treatment of severe depression). But as an alternative or ancillary treatment, I had the right to refuse that therapy. With this experience in mind, I tell parents that while basic psychiatric medications which are FDA-approved for treatment can be administered to their child without their permission, and children will definitely be involved in group counseling sessions, even when in a hospital, a parent will still need to specifically sign waivers of release for any alternative or unusual treatments that are not well-researched or have the risk of potential harmful side-effects. In my clinical experience, even the medication protocols that the treating doctor intends to use are frequently discussed with parents before they are administered to the child. But it is helpful to know that this is not legally required. Essentially, once admitted, the psychiatric doctor on call has the right to recommend medication and therapy in much the same way as the physical health doctor would have the right to treat the patient for a physical illness while in the hospital.

NATUROPATHIC WISDOM

Parents should also know that once placed in a psychiatric hospital neither the individual nor their family can control the timeline for discharge. If there can be a 'silver lining' to a dark situation, unfortunately most hospitals are so 'overfilled' with patients that almost no one is kept longer than is necessary. In fact, I find that for most kids I am involved with, the stay is not long enough. For me personally, I was court-ordered to remain in the hospital for five days. This can happen when the patient (or the patient's parent) disagrees with the discharge timeline and will not consent to stay in the hospital voluntarily beyond seventy-hour hours, or when the threat of suicide or harm to others is severe. My doctor felt that I needed five days on medication for the treatment of depression before I would no longer be an imminent threat to myself. Once in psychiatric care, individuals are frequently court-ordered to remain in the hospital until they are no longer a risk to themselves or others if they attempt to self-discharge too soon.

I will add here that this was the first time in my life that I had been treated for any mental health condition. Prior to this, I had only participated in a few sessions of counseling while in college (which was required for one of my classes), and I had done a handful of sessions with my husband for some marital difficulties. So, when I made the decision to go into the hospital, my family and close friends thought my decision was too extreme. But only I knew how I felt, and I knew I was in real trouble. I also did not trust myself

Chapter 17

to keep ignoring my irrational thoughts. Simply put, I had developed a real desire to end my life, I had established a well-defined plan, I had collected the necessary materials to end my life, and I could no longer give guarantees to those who cared about me that I wouldn't act on my plan 'sometime soon.' When we assess risk for children, these same variables are key in determining the seriousness of a child's intent to harm themselves or others. So, when I talk to a child who knows exactly what they intend to do, their plan is feasible, and they cannot give me a signed written guarantee that they will not act on their plan in the immediate future (I require more than a week), I recommend hospitalization. I might also recommend hospitalization if things are less clear to me, but the child will not self-disclose their thoughts and plans even though they have suggested suicidal ideation, and they seem 'out of it' or despondent. There are several good suicide evaluation services available in most communities, and again, by using the same 988 call number, parents can get professional help in assessing the seriousness of their child or teen's suicidal or violent behavior threats before deciding if hospitalization or a crisis center is necessary.

At the time of my most severe depression, I had also begun monthly injections to suppress my immune system and 'knock down' my white blood cell counts in the hope that these drugs would decrease my allergic reactions. These treatments had made it next to impossible to sleep. In my practice, I have found that any long-term sleep disruption is a red flag for depression and a subsequent mental health crisis. In fact, if a child I am working with is only marginally suicidal (doesn't have a clear plan, doesn't have the means, or doesn't have an immediate desire), if parents can guarantee good, around-the-clock monitoring, I generally recommend that the child take a two- to three-day mental health hiatus from school or other activities to simply wind down and sleep as much as they can. This recommendation comes with limited screen time and few contacts with peers. I'll sometimes also suggest frequent bathing (see chapter on water therapies) and a good nutritional supplement that is in a liquid, easy-to-digest form, along with foods that the child feels are healthy and taste good. In this way, I have kept numerous kids out of the hospital, and by the third day, most kids complain that they are bored, feel better, and want to return to their activities. This method should only be considered when round-the-clock observation can be guaranteed for the child.

In case you do not know this, once placed in psychiatric care, patients also lose their right to communicate freely with family or friends, they are stripped of personal belongings, and in most programs, monitored phone calls and family visits are limited to a certain (and fairly short period of time each day). This too is useful information for both parents and children to know before going in. For me, I was allowed one fifteen-minute phone call and one thirty-minute meeting with my family each day. For children, there are also additional family therapy appointments and meetings with the treating doctors that require parent attendance. But again, while parents can express their opinions about medication and treatment, they have little control over these while their children are hospitalized.

While in the hospital, as I mentioned above, I was treated by a resident psychiatrist who, either by luck or by skilled training, placed me on a standard inpatient psychiatric drug that I later found out also performed as a strong histamine inhibitor; in addition, this medication forced me to sleep. For a full five days, (which felt like a long time), my sleep was punctuated only by three healthy meals, which I was required to eat, a one-hour self-care and breath training class, and three to five hours per day of group therapy. With these experiences, I generally tell my clients that the care their child will receive, if hospitalized, is quite minimal, but with nothing better to do, most patients on an inpatient ward sleep well (even if medicated to do so), eat well (eating three meals a day is required for discharge), and receive some sound, basic mental health instruction along with emergency psychiatric medications.

As terrible as this all sounds, by the time I left the hospital, I genuinely felt lucky to have found a short-term treatment for my depression that amounted to a 'cat-sized dose' of a medication that promoted sleep while also decreasing my inflammatory and histamine responses. I left the hospital with a thirty-day prescription. I also had an appointment (in just ten days) with a psychiatrist that turned out to be exceptionally knowledgeable and helped me a lot in the months that followed with my mental health while I went through some of my early journey towards self-healing. I also learned good things about my breathing patterns and my stress management skills. Last, I left the hospital with an appointment with a therapist (which was required). A commitment to attend counseling and an appointment with a psychiatrist is usually required for discharge, and hospital staff collaborate with the patient and their family to secure these appointments (and help parents jump the line with many psychiatrists) when needed.

As I have looked back on that experience, while it was a really challenging time in my life, I'm glad I can now share it with my clients, when needed, to take some of the fear of the unknown and the stigma out of the inpatient hospitalization experience. Since, I have also come to believe that we all have moments in our lives where we are not very emotionally stable, especially when we are also physically ill. Thus, knowing what to expect if we really need help is important. For the kids I see, especially when talk of self-harm or harming others is present, I also believe we should err on the side of caution. While not every mental health crisis should result in an inpatient psychiatric hospitalization or crisis center, if hospitalization is needed, this can and should be done without fear or shame. I have found that most parents who have had to hospitalize a child feel that the time spent in the hospital was not necessarily that beneficial to their child, but this step was a basic starting point for better psychiatric care in the times that followed.

Final Thoughts and Conclusions

As mentioned above, in addition to taking the unknowns out of mental health crisis treatment, I specifically chose to share this final story because it reminds us to also retain our common sense when it comes to choosing naturopathic over allopathic treatments. Sometimes our kids really are in serious trouble, and during these times, it is not the right time to launch into a host of new naturopathic approaches. Kids who are mentally ill, and in crisis with their illness, must have access to the benefits of evidence-based science with both psychiatry and mental health treatment, just as is true for kids who are critically ill or injured.

As a good rule of thumb, it is safe to say that that all crisis situations (medical or mental health) should be addressed first within allopathic medicine. Without a doubt, allopathic medicine is far superior for treating emergency, critical, and serious health situations. It is also beneficial to remember that naturopathy never treated emergency situations well. In the past, when only naturopathy was available, patients died of their acute injuries, sudden-onset diseases, and illnesses, with at least some of these easily treated today. It should also be clear that naturopathy works slowly and over an extended period of time to return an unhealthy person to a healthier state of stasis and wellness. Naturopathy also does not cure mental illness, just as it does not cure many physical conditions; it is not appropriate for profuse bleeding or broken bones! When we engage with naturopathy appropriately, we must, therefore, dedicate ourselves to the time commitments that real change takes. Schedules, habits, and even lifestyles change when these approaches become a way of life. Last, as a process, naturopathy also requires us to change our views about our self, our health, and our relationship to the planet. For me, there was not an herb or naturopathic treatment within the entire field of naturopathic medicine that could have pulled me out of my severe clinical depression and suicidal ideation, at that time, and in only five short days. In fact, it took years for me to fully treat my depression and my health naturally. For me, this suggests that even if we intend to introduce naturopathy into our practices for education, mental health, or parenting, we need to start first with allopathic practices, especially when the situation is critical. Then, over time, we can slowly introduce naturopathy, beside other treatments for a more long-term and whole-health solution.

I personally do not ever see myself back in the place I was when I started my naturopathic healing journey. But it is not because I expect to stay healthy my whole life. I know I have a deteriorating vertebra, one that is not mine but saved my life that will require another serious surgery in a few short years. I also know that I can easily fall into poor exercise and eating habits from which my hives or seizures might return. I also doubt that I will get through the rest of my life without requiring at least a few prescription medications now and then. The reason I do not ever see myself where I was before is this: my whole attitude about wellness has now changed. I see illness as a way of thinking, I see deep and meaningful connections between physical and mental health, and I see myself in a new, positive, and healthy relationship with the world around me. I also see that rather than feeling helpless about my numerous health challenges, I instead have some enjoyable things I can do to improve my health; this gives me some control over my wellness journey.

This personal and clinical journey of discovery and healthy-minded living brings me to my final statements: 1) kids today seem to need naturopathy more than ever before; 2) pursuing the methods detailed throughout this book need not preclude, exclude, or conclude proper allopathic medical care, as naturopathy is a way of life; 3) as it relates to mental health in children and teens, naturopathic therapies are neither contradicted by nor should they interfere with good mental health or education services; 4) we also needn't feel guilty for choosing one approach over the other, or for going back and forth between these approaches at different periods in our lives; and finally 5) naturopathy is truly a whole-health system that grows into choices and ultimately a lifestyle, which is deeply grounded in the common-sense wisdom of those who have gone before us.

In closing, I hope that we can all strive to find better balance in this fast-paced, evidence-based, sterile world. I believe we can do this through attention to and conscious interaction with the air we breathe, the sun above, the earth's healing waters, the power of human touch, the recuperative power of sleep, and the plants and foods that grow out of the ground beneath our feet. No matter how young or old we are, I also hope that we can take some time to remember a few perfect, still, healing moments in nature from our own childhood, and apply these to our actions today to honor and sustain our planet. I believe that as we interact with our world, we learn from it. Finally, as we more fully explore and discover the healing relationships between our bodies, minds, and our magical earth, I hope we can find ways to bring this wisdom to today's children. Because in the end, the essential principles of naturopathy are the simplest and most basic way that we can live in harmony and health with our world. Living within these basic principles is the basis for deep and complete wellness in both mind and body.

REFERENCES

Ajesh, K. (2018). History of the miasma theory of disease. *ESSAI*, 16(18). Retrieved from https://dc.cod.edu/essai/vol16/iss1/18

Allsopp, M., Visser, S., & Kogan, M. D. (2011). Trends in the prevalence of developmental disabilities in US children, 1997-2008. *Pediatrics*, 127(6), pp. 1034–1042. Retrieved from https://doi.org/10.1542/peds.2010-2989

American Medical Association. (2018). AMA position statement-complementary medicine 2018. *American Medical Association*. Retrieved from https://www.ama.com.au/position-statement/ama-position-statement-complementary-medicine-2018

American Psychiatric Association (APA). (2013). *Diagnostic and statistical manual of mental disorders* (5th ed.). Washington, DC: Author.

Anders, S., & Schroeter, C. (2017). The impact of nutritional supplement intake on diet behavior and obesity outcomes. *PloS One*, 12(10), pp. e0185258. doi.org/10.1371/journal.pone.0185258

Aranow, C. (2012). Vitamin D and the immune system. *Journal of Investigative Medicine: The Official Publication of the American Federation for Clinical Research*, 59(6), pp. 881–886. doi.org/10.2310/JIM.0b013e31821b8755

Ardiel, E. L., & Rankin, C. H. (2010). The importance of touch in development. *Pediatrics & Child Health*, 15(3), pp. 153–156. doi.org/10.1093/pch/15.3.153

Armstrong, T. (2011). *The power of neurodiversity: Unleashing the advantages of your differently wired brain*. Cambridge, MA: Da Capo Press.

Aron, E. N., & Aron, A. (1997). Sensory-processing sensitivity and its relation to introversion and emotionality. *Journal of Personality and Social Psychology*, 73(2), pp. 345–368. doi.org/10.1037//0022-3514.73.2.345

Association of Accredited Naturopathic Medical Colleges (AANMC). (2022). The six principles of naturopathic medicine. Association of Accredited Naturopathic Colleges. Retrieved from https://aanmc.org/6-principles/

Au, D. H., Tsang, H. W., Ling, P. M., Leung, C. H, & Cheung, W. M. (2015). Effects of acupressure on anxiety: A systematic review and meta-analysis. *Acupuncture in Medicine*, 33(5), pp. 353–359. doi:10.1136/acupmed-2014-010720

Aung-Din, R. (2022, May 18). Interview by Thurman, M. P. [Video recording]. Dr. Ron Aung-Din on the use of cannabidiol (CBD) in the treatment of autism, *US Autism Association's Online Video Library*, West Hartford, CT.

Avena, N. M., & Hoebel, B. G. (2012). Binging, withdrawal, and craving: An animal model of sugar addiction, in Kelly D. Brownell, and Mark S. Gold (eds), *Food and addiction: A comprehensive handbook*, New York, NY: Oxford Academic. Retrieved from https:/0/doi.org/10.1093/med:psych/9780199738168.003.0031.

Ayers, J. (1979). *Sensory integration and the child*. Los Angeles: Western Psychological Services.

References

Ayers, J. A. (1972). Improving academic scores through sensory integration. *Journal of Learning Disabilities*, 5, pp. 338–343. doi.org/10.1177/002221947200500605

Babar, A., Naser, A., Wabel, S. Aftab, A., Shah, A. K., and Firoz, A. (2015). Essential oils used in aromatherapy: A systemic review. *Asian Pacific Journal of Tropical Biomedicine*,5(8), pp. 601-611. doi.org/10.1016/j.apjtb.2015.05.007

Bakke, A. J., Shehan, C. V., & Hayes, J. E. (2016). Type of milk typically consumed, and stated preference, but not health consciousness effect revealed preferences for fat in milk. *Food Quality and Preference*, 49, pp. 92–99. doi.org/10.1016/j.foodqual.2015.12.001

Bakley, S. (2001). Through the lens of sensory integration: A different way of analyzing challenging behavior. *Young Children*, 56(6), pp. 70-76. Retrieved from https://eric.ed.gov/?id=EJ652626

Barker, A.L. Talevski, J., Morello, R. T., Brand, C. A., Rahmann, A. E., & Urquhart, D. (2014). Effectiveness of aquatic exercise for musculoskeletal conditions: A meta-analysi, *Archives of Physical Medicine and Rehabilitation*, 95 (9), pp. 1776–1786, doi.org/10.1016/j.apmr.2014.04.005.

Bates, L. C, Zieff, G., Stanford, K., Moore, J. B, Kerr, Z. Y., Hanson E. D., Barone Gibbs, B., Kline, C. E., & Stoner, L. (2020). COVID-19 impact on behaviors across the 24-hour day in children and adolescents: Physical activity, sedentary behavior, and sleep. *Children*. 7(9), p. 138. doi.org/10.3390/children7090138

Becker, M., & Correll, C. U. (2020). Suicidality in Childhood and Adolescence. *Deutsches Arzteblatt International*, 117(15), pp. 261–267. doi.org/10.3238/arztebl.2020.0261

Benjamin, P. Tappan, F. (2005) *Handbook of healing massage techniques* Upper Saddle River, NJ: Pearson Prentice Hall,

Blaikie, N. (2007). *Approaches to social enquiry: Advancing knowledge.* Cambridge, MA: Polity Press.

Blume, C., Garbazza, C., & Spitschan, M. (2019). Effects of light on human circadian rhythms, sleep, and mood. *Sleep Research and Sleep Medicine*, 23(3), pp. 147–156. doi.org/10.1007/s11818-019-00215-x

Bordley, J. A. and McGehee, H. (1976). *Two centuries of American medicine, 1776–1976.* Philadelphia, PA: Saunders.

Boyle, C. A., Boulet, S., Schieve, L. A., Cohen, R. A., Blumberg, S. J., Yeargin-Allsopp, M., ... & Kogan, M. D. (2011). Trends in the prevalence of developmental disabilities in US children, 1997–2008. *Pediatrics*, 127(6), pp. 1034-1042 doi.org/10.1542/peds.2010-2989

Briar, B. (2019, October 20). Ancient Egyptian creation myths: Of water and gods. *Wondrium Daily*, Retrieved from https://www.wondriumdaily. com/ancient-egyptian-creation-myths-of-water-and-gods/

Britannica, T. Editors of Encyclopedia (2021, May 9). *Germ theory. Encyclopedia Britannica.* Retrieved from https://www.britannica.com/science/germ-theory

Burr, V. (2003). *Social constructionism.* New York, NY: Routledge.

Buzan, T. & Buzan, B. (1993). *The Mind Map Book.* London: BBC Books.

Carissa J., Cascio, D., Moore, F. M., (2019). Social touch and human development, *Developmental Cognitive Neuroscience*, 35(5), pp. 5–11. doi. org/10.1016/j.dcn.2018.04.009

References

Castelli, D. M., Hillman, C. H., Buck, S. M., & Erwin, H. E. (2007). Physical fitness and academic achievement in third- and fifth-grade students. *Journal of Sport & Exercise Psychology*, 29(2), pp. 239–252. doi.org/10.1123/jsep.29.2.239

Centers for Disease Control (CDC). (2021, December). Prevalence and Characteristics of Autism Spectrum Disorder Among Children—Autism and Developmental Disabilities Monitoring Network, *Surveillance Summaries*, 70 (11), pp. 1–16 Retrieved from https://www.cdc.gov/mmwr/volumes/70/ss/ss7011a1.htm

Centers for Disease Control (CDC). (2022, November). Data and Statistics on Children's Mental Health. *Children's Mental Health*, retrieved from https://www.cdc.gov/childrensmentalhealth/data.html

Chen, W, Faris MAE, Bragazzi NL, AlGahtani HMS, Saif Z, Jahrami A, Shivappa N, Hebert JR, Jahrami H. (2021, April). Diet-related inflammation is associated with major depressive disorder: Results of a case-control study using the Dietary Inflammatory Index. *Journal of Inflammatory Research*; 14:1, pp. 437-1445. doi:10.2147/JIR.S306315

Chen, C. W., Tai, C. J., Choy, C. S., Hsu, C. Y., Lin, S. L., Chan, W. P., Chiang, H. S., Chen, C. A., & Leung, T. K. (2013). Wave-induced flow in meridians demonstrated using photoluminescent bioceramic material on acupuncture points. *Evidence-Based Complementary and Alternative Medicine:eCAM*, 2013, 739293. doi.org/10.1155/2013/739293

Children's Hospital of Philadelphia. (2022, March). Aromatherapy for children: What's safe and what's not. *Integrative Health*. Retrieved from https://www.chop.edu/news/health-tip/aromatherapy-children-whats-safe-and-whats-not

Chung, L. M. Y., & Fong, S. S. M. (2018). Appearance alteration of fruits and vegetables to increase their appeal to and consumption by school-age children: A pilot study. *Health Psychology Open*, 5(2), pp. 2055102918802679. doi.org/10.1177/2055102918802679

Cody, G. W. (2018). The Origins of Integrative Medicine-The First True Integrators: The Philosophy of Early Practitioners. *Integrative medicine*, 17(2), pp. 16–18. Retrieved from https://www.ncbi.nlm.nih.gov/pmc/articles/PMC6396756/

Cutler, E. (2010). *The food allergy cure: A new solution to food cravings, obesity, depression, headaches, arthritis, and fatigue.* New York, NY: Harmony.

Czeranko, S. (2019). Pioneers of Naturopathic Medicine. *Integrative Medicine*, 18(4), p. 40. Retrieved from https://www.ncbi.nlm.nih.gov/pmc/articles/PMC7219465/

Denver Post. (2020, August 6). Home Depot Told to Pay. Retrieved from https://extras.denverpost.com/news/news0806p.htm

de Souza, R. G. M., Schincaglia, R. M., Pimentel, G. D., & Mota, J. F. (2017). Nuts and Human Health Outcomes: A Systematic Review. *Nutrients*, 9(12), p. 311. doi.org/10.3390/nu9121311

Dhabhar F. S. (2018). The short-term stress response - Mother nature's mechanism for enhancing protection and performance under conditions of threat, challenge, and opportunity. *Frontiers in Neuroendocrinology*, 49, pp. 175–192. doi.org/10.1016/j.yfrne.2018.03.004

DiMatties, M. E. & Sammons, J. H. (2003). *Understanding sensory integration* (ED478564). Arlington VA: ERIC Clearinghouse on Disabilities and Gifted Education.

Dossett, M. L., & Yeh, G. Y. (2018). Homeopathy use in the United States and implications for public health: A review. *Homeopathy: The Journal of the Faculty of Homeopathy*, 107(1), pp. 3–9. doi.org/10.1055/s-0037-1609016

References

Eysenck, M. W. & Calvo, M. G. (1997). Anxiety and performance: The proceessing efficiency theory. *Cognition and Emotion*, 6, pp. 409–434. doi. org/10.1080/02699939208409696

Faria M. A., Jr (2013). Violence, mental illness, and the brain - A brief history of psychosurgery: Part 1 - From trephination to lobotomy. *Surgical Neurology International*, 4 (49). doi.org/10.4103/2152-7806.110146

Farr, A., Curlin, K., Rasinski, T., et. al. (2009). Clinicians and the integration of complementary and alternative medicines. *The Journal of Alternative and Complimentary Medicine*, 15(9), pp. 987-994. doi.org/10.1089/acm.2008.0512

Fee, E. (2015). The First American Medical Schools: The Formative Years. The Lancet, 385(9981), pp.1940–1941. Retrieved from https://www.thelancet.com/journals/lancet/article/PIIS0140-6736(15)60950-3/fulltext

Finkelhor, D. (2010). Child sex abuse statistics. *National Center for Victims of Crime*. Retrieved from https://victimsofcrime.org/child-sexual-abuse-statistics/

Food Research Action Center. (2022). Hunger and poverty in America. *White House Conference on Hunger*. Retrieved from https://frac.org/hunger-poverty-america

Fuller, C., Lehman, E., Hicks, S., & Novick, M. B. (2017). Bedtime use of technology and associated sleep problems in children. *Global Pediatric Health*, 4, 2333794X17736972. doi.org/10.1177/2333794X17736972

Getz, M., Hutzler. Y., & Vermeer, A. Effects of aquatic interventions in children with neuromotor impairments: a systematic review of the literature. *Clinical Rehabilitation*, 20(11), pp. 927–936. doi:10.1177/0269215506070693

NATUROPATHIC WISDOM

Gianfaldoni, S., Tchernev, G., Wollina, U., Roccia, M. G., Fioranelli, M., Gianfaldoni, R., & Lotti, T. (2017). History of the baths and thermal medicine. *Open Access Macedonian Journal of Medical Sciences*, 5(4), pp. 566–568. doi.org/10.3889/oamjms.2017.126

Gürol, S., Polat, S. (2012). The effects of baby massage on attachment between mothers and their Infants, *Asian Nursing Research*, 6(1), pp. 35–41. doi.org/10.1016/j.anr.2012.02.006

Hansotia, P. (2003). A neurologist looks at mind and brain: "The enchanted loom." *Clinical Medicine and Research*, 1(4), pp. 327–332. Retrieved from https://www.ncbi.nlm.nih.gov/pmc/articles/PMC1069062/

Higgins, T. R., Greene, D. A., Baker, M. K. (2017). Effects of cold-water immersion and contrast water therapy for recovery from team sport: A systematic review and meta-analysis. *Journal of Strength and Conditioning Research*, 31(5), pp. 1443–1460. Retrieved from https://journals.lww.com/nsca-jscr/Fulltext/2017/05000/Effects_of_Cold_Water_Immersion_and_Contrast_Water.32.aspx

Holland, B. (2019, April). 7 of the most outrageous medical treatments in history, *History*, Retrieved from https://www.history.com/news/7-of-the-most-outrageous-medical-treatments-in-history

Hussain, J., & Cohen, M. (2018). Clinical effects of regular dry sauna bathing: A systematic review. *Evidence-Based Complementary and Alternative Medicine: eCAM*, 2018, doi.org/10.1155/2018/1857413

Jiyeon, A. Lee, I., & Yi, Y. (2019) The thermal effects of water immersion on health outcomes: An integrative review. *International Journal of Environmental Research and Public Health* 16(7), pp. 1280. doi.org/10.3390/ijerph16071280

References

Katiyar, C., Gupta, A., Kanjilal, S., & Katiyar, S. (2012). Drug discovery from plant sources: An integrated approach. *Ayu*, 33(1), pp. 10–19. doi.org/10.4103/0974-8520.100295

Kenyan, J. (1988). *Acupressure techniques: Well-being and pain relief at your fingertips*. Manhattan, NY: Healing Arts Press.

Knowles, R. (2022, April 2). Interview by Thurman, M. P [Video Recording] How bottom-up therapies can mitigate meltdowns and neuro-cashes. US Autism Association's Online Video Library, West Hartford, CT.

Ko, Y. (2016). Sebastian Kneipp and the natural cure movement of Germany: Between naturalism and modern medicine. *Ui Sahak*, 25(3), pp. 557–590. doi.org/10.13081/kjmh.2016.25.557

Lagay, F. (2002). The legacy of humoral medicine. *American Medical Association Journal of Ethics*, 4(7), pp. 206–208. Retrieved from https://journalofethics.ama-assn.org/article/legacy-humoral-medicine/2002-07

Lambourne, K., Audiffren, M., & Tomporowski, P. D. (2010). Effects of acute exercise on sensroy and executive processing tasks. *Medicine and Science in Sports and Exercise*, 4, pp. 1396–1402. Retrieved from https://www.researchgate.net/publication/40696924_Effects_of_Acute_Exercise_on_Sensory_and_Executive_Processing_

Let Nature Take Its Course (idiom). (2022). In *Merriam-Webster's online dictionary* (11th ed.). Retrieved from https://www.merriam-webster.com/dictionary/let%20nature%20take%20its%20course

Li, Q. (2018, May) Forest bathing is great for your health. Here's how to do it. *Time, Live Well Division*. Retrieved from: https://time.com/5259602/japanese-forest-bathing/

Lin, D., Xiao, M., Zhao, J., Li, Z., Xing, B., Li, X., Kong, M., Li, L., Zhang, Q., Liu, Y., Chen, H., Qin, W., Wu, H., & Chen, S. (2016). An overview of plant phenolic compounds and their importance in human nutrition and management of type 2 diabetes. *Molecules*, 21(10), p. 1374. doi.org/10.3390/molecules21101374

Liu, A. G., Ford, N. A., Hu, F. B., Zelman, K. M., Mozaffarian, D., & Kris-Etherton, P. M. (2017). A healthy approach to dietary fats: understanding the science and taking action to reduce consumer confusion. *Nutrition Journal*, 16(1), p. 53. doi.org/10.1186/s12937-017-0271-4

Locher, C., & Pforr, C. (2014). The legacy of Sebastian Kneipp: linking wellness, naturopathic, and allopathic medicine. *Journal of Alternative and Complementary Medicine*, 20(7), pp. 521–526. doi.org/10.1089/acm.2013.042

MacMillan, C. (2022, August 1). Is my sunscreen safe? Recent reports link certain sunscreens to cancer-causing chemicals. *Yale Medicine Online News*. Retrieved from https://www.yalemedicine.org/news/is-sunscreen-safe

Mandal, S. M., Chakraborty, D., & Dey, S. (2010). Phenolic acids act as signaling molecules in plant-microbe symbioses. *Plant Signaling & Behavior*, 5(4), pp. 359–368. doi.org/10.4161/psb.5.4.10871

March, R. J. & Geloso, V. (2020). Gordon Tullock meets Phineas Gage: The political economy of lobotomies in the United States. *Research Policy*, 49(1). doi.org/10.1016/j.respol.2019.103872

McMahon, W. M., & Ritvo, A. (1989). The UCLA-University of Utah epidemiologic survey of autism prevalence. *American Journal of Psychiatry*, 146(2), pp. 194–199. Retrieved from http://citeseerx.ist.psu.edu/viewdoc/download?doi=10.1.1.456.4606&rep=rep1&type=pdf

References

McRae, M. P. (2017). Health benefits of dietary whole grains: An umbrella review of meta-analyses. *Journal of Chiropractic Medicine*, 16(1), pp. 10–18. doi.org/10.1016/j.jcm.2016.08.008

Mead, M. N. (2008). Benefits of sunlight: a bright spot for human health. *Environmental Health Perspectives*, 116(4), pp. A160–A167. doi.org/10.1289/ehp.116-a160

Medawar, E., Huhn, S., Villringer, A., & Veronica Witte, A. (2019). The effects of plant-based diets on the body and the brain: a systematic review. *Translational Psychiatry*, 9(1), p. 226. doi.org/10.1038/s41398-019-0552-0

Medeiros, M. F., de Albuquerque, U. P. (2012). The pharmacy of the Benedictine monks. *Journal of Ethnopharmacology*, 139 (1), pp. 280-286. Retrieved from https://www.sciencedirect.com/science/article/pii/S0378874111008129

Meier, Christine (2022, October). Forest bathing, the Japanese therapy approach. *Mibelle Biochemistry Group*. Retrieved from https://mibellebio-chemistry.com/forest-bathing-japanese-therapy-approach

Mennella, J. A., & Bobowski, N. K. (2015). The sweetness and bitterness of childhood: Insights from basic research on taste preferences. *Physiology & Behavior*, 152 (Pt B), pp. 502–507. doi.org/10.1016/j.physbeh.2015.05.015

Merriam, S. B.. (2009). *Qualitative research: A guide to design and implementation*. San Francisco, CA: Jossey-Bass.

Merriam, S. B., & Tisdell, E. J. (2015). *Qualitative research: A guide to design and implementation*. Hoboken, NJ: John Wiley & Sons.

Metzgar, D. (2022, November 1). What is touch therapy and why your kid might need it. *Parents*. Retrieved from: https://www.parents.com/kids/health/what-is-touch-therapy-and-why-your-kid-might-need-it/

Michealides, D. (Eds). (2014). *Medicine and healing in the ancient Mediterranean world*. Oxford, UK: Oxbow Books

Migala, J. (2022, January 10). *U.S. News and World Report* reveals best and worst diets of 2022. *U.S. News and World Report*. Retrieved from https://www.everydayhealth.com/diet-and-nutrition/diet/us-news-best-diet-plans-mediterranean-dash-more/

Miyazaki, Y. (2022, May 3). Interview by Thurman, M. P. [Video recording]. Shinrin-yoku: The art and science of forest bathing]. *US Autism Association's Online Video Library*, West Hartford, CT.

Mortimer, R., Privopoulos, M., & Kumar, S. (2014). The effectiveness of hydrotherapy in the treatment of social and behavioral aspects of children with autism spectrum disorders: a systematic review. *Journal of Multidisciplinary Healthcare*, 7, pp. 93–104. doi.org/10.2147/JMDH.S55345

Moss GA. (2010). Water and health: A forgotten connection? *Perspectives in Public Health*. 130(5), pp. 227-232. doi:10.1177/1757913910379192

Moyer, C. A., Rounds, J., & Hannum, J. W. (2004). A meta-analysis of massage therapy research. *Psychological Bulletin*, 130(1), pp. 3–18. doi.org/10.1037/0033-2909.130.1.

Mullin, G. E., & Dobs, A. (2007). Vitamin D and its role in cancer immunity: A prescription for sunlight. *Nutrition in Clinical Practice*. doi.org/10.1177/0115426507022003305

Myers, J. P., Antoniou, M. N., Blumberg, B., Carroll, L., Colborn, T., Everett, L. G., Hansen, M., Landrigan, P. J., Lanphear, B. P., Mesnage, R.,

References

Vandenberg, L. N., Vom Saal, F. S., Welshons, W. V., & Benbrook, C. M. (2016). Concerns over use of glyphosate-based herbicides and risks associated with exposures: a consensus statement. *Environmental Health : A Global Access Science Source*, 15, 19. doi.org/10.1186/s12940-016-0117-0

Newson, L. P. (2006). Medical practice in early colonial Spanish America: A prospectus. *Bulletin of Latin American Research* ,5(3), pp. 367–391. Retrieved from https://www.academia.edu/ 26306242/Medical_Practice_in_Early_Colonial_Spanish_ America_A_Prospectus

New York Society for the Prevention of Cruelty to Children (2022, November 1). *What is Safe Touches?* New York: NY, Author. Retrieved from https:// nyspcc.org/what-we-do/training-institute/professional-trainings-and-resources/safe-touches/

Oakenfull, D., & Sidhu, G. S. (1992). Low-Cholesterol Egg and Dairy Products. *Outlook on Agriculture*, 21(3), pp. 203–208. doi.org/10.1177/003072709202100309

Pall, M. L. (2009). Do sauna therapy and exercise act by raising the availability of tetrahydrobiopterin? *Medical Hypotheses*,73 (4), pp. 610-613. doi.org/10.1016/j.mehy.2009.03.058

Pan, S. Y., Litscher, G., Gao, S. H., Zhou, S. F., Yu, Z. L., Chen, H. Q., Zhang, S. F., Tang, M. K., Sun, J. N., & Ko, K. M. (2014). Historical perspective of traditional indigenous medical practices: the current renaissance and conservation of herbal resources. *Evidence-Based Complementary and Alternative Medicine*. Retrieved from https://pubmed.ncbi.nlm.nih.gov/782235/

Panos, M. B. & Heimlich, J. (1980). *Homeopathic medicine at home*. New York, NY: Penguin Publications.

NATUROPATHIC WISDOM

Parascandola J. (1976). Drug therapy in colonial and revolutionary America. *American Journal of Hospital Pharmacy*, 33(8), pp. 807–810. Retrieved from https://pubmed.ncbi.nlm.nih.gov/782235/

Phillips, S. R., Johnson, A. H., Shirey, M. R., & Rice, M. (2020). Sleep quality in school-aged children: A concept analysis. *Journal of Pediatric Nursing*, 52, pp. 54–63. doi.org/10.1016/j.pedn.2020.02.043

Ponzo, V., Pellegrini, M., Costelli, P., Vázquez-Araújo, L., Gayoso, L., D'Eusebio, C., Ghigo, E., & Bo, S. (2021). Strategies for reducing salt and sugar intake in individuals at increased cardiometabolic risk. *Nutrients*, 13(1), p. 279. doi.org/10.3390/nu13010279

Racine, N., McArthur, B.A., Cooke, J.E., Eirich, R., Zhu, J., & Madigan, S. (2021). Global prevalence of mental health symptoms in children and adolescents: A meta-analysis. *Journal of American Pediatrics*, 175(11), pp. 1142–115. doi:10.1001/jamapediatrics.2021.2482.

Rajaei, S., Kalantari, M., Pashazadeh Azari, Z., Tabatabaee, S. M., & Dunn, W. (2020). Sensory processing patterns and sleep quality in primary school children. *Iranian Journal of Child Neurology*, 14(3), pp. 57–68. Retrieved from https://www.ncbi.nlm.nih.gov/pmc/articles/PMC7468082/

Rasoanaivo, P., Wright, C. W., Willcox, M. L., & Gilbert, B. (2011). Whole plant extracts versus single compounds for the treatment of malaria: synergy and positive interactions. *Malaria Journal*, 10 Suppl 1 (Suppl 1), S4. doi.org/10.1186/1475-2875-10-S1-S4

Richi, E. B., Baumer, B., Conrad, B., Darioli, R., Schmid, A., & Keller, U. (2015). Health risks associated with meat consumption: a review of epidemiological studies. *International Journal of Nutrition Research*, 85(1-2), pp. 70–78. Retrieved from https://www.researchgate.net/profile/Ulrich-Keller2/publication/324197541_Aspects_sanitaires_de_la_consommation_

References

de_viande/links/5e8ae65792851c2f5282d6ca/Aspects-sanitaires-de-la-consommation-de-viande.pdf

Relton, C., Cooper, K., Viksveen, P., Fibert, P., & Thomas, K. (2017). Prevalence of homeopathy use by the general population worldwide: a systematic review. *Homeopathy: The Journal of the Faculty of Homeopathy*, 106(2), pp. 69–78. doi.org/10.1016/j.homp.2017.03.002

Reiley, L. (2019, October 17). Sweet excess: How the baby food industry hooks toddlers on sugar, salt, and fat. *Washington Post*. Retrieved from https://www.washingtonpost.com/business/2019/10/17/sweet-excess-how-baby-food-industry-hooks-toddlers-sugar-salt-fat/https://doi.org/10.1542/peds.2006-2089F

Rew, L., Young, C., Harrison, T., & Caridi, R. (2015). A systematic review of literature on psychosocial aspects of gynecomastia in adolescents and young men. *Journal of Adolescence*, 43, pp. 206–212. doi.org/10.1016/j.adolescence.2015.06.007

Smaldone, A., Honig, J. C., & Byrne, M. W. (2007). Sleepless in America: Inadequate sleep and relationships to health and well-being of our nation's children. *Pediatrics*, 119 (1), pp. S29–S37. doi.org/10.1542/peds.2006-2089F

Smith, B. J., Grunseit, A., Hardy, L. L., King, L., Wolfenden, L., & Milat, A. (2010). Parental influences on child physical activity and screen viewing time: a population-based study. *BMC Public Health*, 10(1), pp. 1–11. Retrieved from https://link.springer.com/content/pdf/10.1186/1471-2458-10-593.pdf

Snider, P., & Zeff, J. (2019). Unifying Principles of Naturopathic Medicine *Origins and Definitions. Integrative Medicine*, 18(4), pp. 36–39. Retrieved from https://www.ncbi.nlm.nih.gov/pmc/articles/PMC7219457/

Soemarie, Y. B., Milanda, T., & Barliana, M. I. (2021). Fermented foods as probiotics: A review. *Journal of Advanced Pharmaceutical Technology & Research*, 12(4), pp. 335–339. doi.org/10.4103/japtr.japtr_116_21

Starr, P. (2004). The social transformation of American medicine. *Journal of Health and Political Policy Law*, 29 (4-5), pp. 575–620. doi.org/10.1215/03616878-29-4-5-575

Steinemann, A. (2016). Fragranced consumer products: exposures and effects from emissions. *Air Quality, Atmosphere, & Health*, 9(8), pp. 861–866. doi.org/10.1007/s11869-016-0442-z

Stiglic, N., & Viner, R. M. (2019). Effects of screentime on the health and well-being of children and adolescents: a systematic review of reviews. *BMJ Open*, 9(1), p. e023191. Retrieved from https://bmjopen.bmj.com/content/bmjopen/9/1/e023191.full.pdf

Sugar substitutes: Health controversy over perceived benefits. *Journal of Pharmacology & Pharmacotherapeutics*, 2(4), pp. 236–243. doi.org/10.4103/0976-500X.85936.

Paulien, G. B. (1995). *The divine prescription and science of health and healing*. Brushton, NY: TEACH Services Inc.

Saturni, L., Ferretti, G., & Bacchetti, T. (2010). The gluten-free diet: safety and nutritional quality. *Nutrients*, 2(1), pp. 16–34. doi.org/10.3390/nu20100016

Schaaf, R. C., & Miller, L. J. (2005). Occupational therapy using a sensory integrative approach for children with developmental disabilities. *Mental Retardation and Developmental Disabilities Research Reviews*, 11(2), pp. 143–148. doi.org/10.1002/mrdd.20067

References

Shacher, C. & Reiss, D. R. (2020). When are vaccine mandates appropriate. *AMA Journal of Ethics* 22(1), pp, e36–42. doi:10.1001/amajethics.2020.36.

Sharps, J. (1995). *Basic principles of total health.* Smithfield, Virginia: International Institute of Original Medicine.

Sharps, E. Sharps, J. Turley, S. (2010) *Ways to wellness.* Smithfield, Virginia: International Institute of Original Medicine.

Shelton, H. M. (2010). *Human life, its philosophy, and laws: An exposition of the principles and practices of orthopathy.* Whitefish, Montana: Kessinger Legacy Reprints.

Shook, E., (1992). *Advanced treatise in herbology.* Banning, CA: Enos Publishing

Sirajudeen, S., Shah, I., & Al Menhali, A. (2019). A narrative role of vitamin D and its receptor: With current evidence on the gastric tissues. *International Journal of Molecular Sciences*, 20(15), p. 3832. doi.org/10.3390/ijms20153832n

Smith K. A. (2012). Louis Pasteur, the father of immunology? *Frontiers in Immunology*, 3, 68. doi.org/10.3389/fimmu.2012.00068

Stewart, D. (2016) *The chemistry of essential oils made simple*: Marble Hill, MO: Care Publications.

Stromberg, J. (2013, April). What's in century-old 'snake oil' medicines? *Smithsonian Magazine*. Retrieved from https://www.smithsonianmag.com/science-nature/whats-in-century-old-snake-oil-medicines-mercury-and-lead-16743639/

Tesh S. (1981). Disease causality and politics. *Journal of Health Politics, Policy, and Law*, 6(3), pp. 369–390. doi.org/10.1215/03616878-6-3-369

Theberath, M., Bauer, D., Chen, W., Salinas, M., Mohabbat, A. B., Yang, J., Chon, T. Y., Bauer, B. A., & Wahner-Roedler, D. L. (2022). Effects of COVID-19 pandemic on mental health of children and adolescents: A systematic review of survey studies. *SAGE Open Medicine*, 10, 20503121221086712.

Thiel, R. (2000) *Naturopathy for the 21ˢᵗ century*. Warsaw, IN: Whitman Publications

Trochim, W., & Donnelly, J. (2001). *Research methods knowledge base*. Ithaca, New York: Cornell University.

Tsitsis, N, Polkas, G., Daoutis, G., & Prokopiou, A. (2013). Hydrotherapy in ancient Greece. *Balkan Military Medical Review*, 16 (4), pp. 462-466. Retrieved from https://www.researchgate.net/publication/298335209_Hydrotherapy_in_Ancient_Greece

Unulu, M. & Nurten, K. (2017). The effect of neiguan point (P6) acupressure with wristband on postoperative nausea, vomiting, and comfort level: A randomized controlled study, *Journal of Perianesthesia Nursing: Official Journal of the American Society of PeriAnesthesia Nurses / American Society of PeriAnesthesia Nurses*, 33(6), Retrieved from https://www.researchgate.net/publication/320848634_The_Effect_of_Neiguan_Point_P6_Acupressure_With_Wristband_on_Postoperative_Nausea_Vomiting_and_Comfort_Level_A_Randomized_Controlled_Study

U.S. Department of Education, (2004). *Building the legacy: IDEA 2004*. Retrieved from http://idea.ed.gov

van Tubergen, A., & van der Linden, S. (2002). A brief history of spa therapy. *Annals of the Rheumatic diseases*, 61(3), pp. 273–275. doi. org/10.1136/ard.61.3.273

References

Wacker, M., & Holick, M. F. (2013). Sunlight and vitamin D: A global perspective for health. *Dermato-Endocrinology*, 5(1), pp. 51–108. doi. org/10.4161/derm.24494

Watson, M., Holman, D. M., & Maguire-Eisen, M. (2016). Ultraviolet radiation exposure and its impact on skin cancer risk. *Seminars in Oncology Nursing*, 32(3), pp. 241–254. doi.org/10.1016/j.soncn.2016.05.005

White, E. (1976). *Counsels on Diet and Food*, Hagerstown, MD: Review and Herald Publishing Association.

White, J. R., Jr. (2018). Sugar. *Clinical Diabetes: A Publication of the American Diabetes Association*, 36(1), pp. 74–76. doi.org/10.2337/cd17-0084

Wilcock, I. M., Cronin, J. B., & Hing, W. A. (2006). Physiological response to water immersion. *Sports Medicine*, 36(9), pp, 747-765. doi.org/10.3390/ijerph16071280

Winter, C. K., & Katz, J. M. (2011). Dietary exposure to pesticide residues from commodities alleged to contain the highest contamination levels. *Journal of Toxicology*, 589674. doi.org/10.1155/2011/589674

Wiss, D. A., Avena, N., & Rada, P. (2018). Sugar addiction: From evolution to revolution. *Frontiers in Psychiatry*, 9, p. 545. doi.org/10.3389/fpsyt.2018.00545

Wolfe, R. M., & Sharp, L. K. (2002). Anti-vaccinationists past and present. *BMJ*, 325(7361), pp. 430-432. doi.org/10.1136/bmj.325.7361.430

Yilmaz, I., Yanardag, M., Birkan, B., & Bumin, G. (2004). Effects of swimming training on physical fitness and water orientation in autism. *Pediatrics International*, 46(5), pp. 624–626. doi.org/10.1111/J.1442-200X.2004.01938.X

AUTHOR BIO

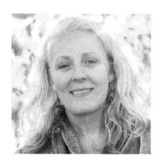

Marlo Payne Thurman, PhD, began her career in 1992 as a private practice school psychologist. Through the years she has held positions with various group homes, mental health centers, hospital clinics, and schools in conjunction with providing assessment, advocacy, consultation, and counseling services in her practice to thousands of clients. For ten years she also owned and ran a special needs private school that made national headlines for successfully serving twice-exceptional students. She is also the author of *Autism Is the Future: The Evolution of a Different Type of Intelligence*. She is currently the President and Board Chair of the U.S. Autism Association. Always dividing her time between her private practice work, continuing education, and various charity endeavors, Marlo made the decision to pursue a final degree in the field of naturopathic medicine. This book is the culmination of that degree, as it combines her history, her personal wellness journey, and her remarkable insights as both an educator and mental health practitioner. Marlo lives in Colorado where she is an avid outdoor enthusiast and gardener.

Printed in the USA
CPSIA information can be obtained
at www.ICGtesting.com
JSHW011111010524
62269JS00004B/6